Hyperthermia in Oncology – Principles and Therapeutic Outlook

UNI-MED

UNI-MED Verlag AG
Bremen - London - Boston

Ott, Oliver:
Hyperthermia in Oncology – Principles and Therapeutic Outlook/Oliver J. Ott, Rolf D. Issels, Rüdiger Wessalowski.-
2nd edition - Bremen: UNI-MED, 2024
(UNI-MED SCIENCE)
ISBN 978-3-8374-1665-7

Printed in Europe

MEDICINE - STATE OF THE ART

UNI-MED Verlag AG, one of the leading medical publishing companies in Germany, presents its highly successful series of scientific textbooks, covering all medical subjects. The authors are specialists in their fields and present the topics precisely, comprehensively, and with the facility of quick reference in mind. The books will be most useful for all doctors who wish to keep up to date with the latest developments in medicine.

Preface and acknowledgements

During the past decade clinical evidence on the beneficial use of additive local and regional hyperthermia procedures as part of multimodality treatment approaches for several malignant diseases has increased significantly. With the publication of relevant clinical trials and analyses, additive local and regional hyperthermia procedures regained attention globally among oncological professionals and its potential beneficial effect is described in several guidelines. Therefore, the evidence-based use of hyperthermia treatments is reimbursed by health insurances in various countries. Today, hyperthermia plays a role in the treatment of chest wall recurrences after breast cancer, locally advanced cervical cancer, locally advanced and recurrent rectal cancer, high risk soft tissue sarcoma, anal carcinoma and bladder cancer.

Recent technical advances are contributing to improved quality assurance. With the help of CT- or MRI-based planning systems, the temperature distribution in the target area can be preplanned and optimized before the patient is exposed, and in the clinical setting, the calculated heat distribution can be verified with a dedicated MRI scanner for non-invasive thermometry. Meanwhile, hyperthermia treatment quality assurance and delivery standards had been improved and published by a dedicated team of physicists, technicians and clinicians.

This booklet is dedicated to the interested reader without any expertise in local and regional hyperthermia. It is designed to provide instant access: The first part of the book gives a compact overview on the definition of hyperthermia, the physical mode of action for controlled tissue heating, and the biological effects associated with hyperthermia. In the second part, hyperthermia procedures and clinical indications are described and practical recommendations for the treatment delivery and quality assurance are given. In the third part, clinical results for the combined use of hyperthermia with radio- and/or chemotherapy are summarized. A special spotlight is set on the role of hyperthermia in the treatment of childhood malignancies. This part of the booklet is completed with the presentation of currently open or future clinical trials.

We hope that the interested reader will enjoy reading and will get fast access and understanding for the potential of quality-assured local and regional hyperthermia procedures in combination with oncological standard treatments.

Erlangen, January 2024

Oliver J. Ott
Rolf D. Issels
Rüdiger Wessalowski

Authors

Editors

Prof. Dr. med. Oliver J. Ott (Editor)
Dept. of Radiation Oncology
University Hospital Erlangen
Universitätsstraße 27
91054 Erlangen
Germany

Chapters 2.1., 3.1., 3.3., 3.4., 5.2., 6.

Prof. Dr. med. Dipl.-Biochem. Rolf D. Issels (Co-Editor)
Dept. of Medicine III
LMU University Hospital
LMU Munich
Marchioninistraße 15
81377 Munich
Germany

and

Helmholtz Zentrum München
Institute of Molecular Immunology
CCG Hyperthermia
Marchioninistraße 25
81377 Munich
Germany

Chapters 3.2., 5.1., 6.

Priv. Doz. Dr. med. Rüdiger Wessalowski (Co-Editor)
Dept. of Pediatric Oncology, Hematology and Clinical Immunology
University Hospital Düsseldorf
Moorenstraße 5
40225 Düsseldorf
Germany

Chapters 4., 6.

Co-authors

Dipl.-Ing. Sultan Abdel-Rahman
Dept. of Medicine III
LMU University Hospital
LMU Munich
Marchioninistraße 15
81377 Munich
Germany

Chapter 2.2.

Prof. Dr. rer. nat. habil. Udo S. Gaipl
Dept. of Radiation Oncology
Translational Radiobiology
University Hospital Erlangen
Universitätsstraße 27
91054 Erlangen
Germany

Chapter 1.3.

Dr. rer. nat. Andreas Jordan
MagForce NT GmbH
Max-Planck-Straße 3
12489 Berlin
Germany

Chapter 2.1.

Univ.-Prof. Dr. med. Lars H. Lindner
Dept. of Medicine III
LMU University Hospital
LMU Munich
Marchioninistraße 15
81377 Munich
Germany

Chapters 2.1., 2.2, 3.2., 5.1.

Dr. med. Valeria Milani
Dept. of Medicine III
LMU University Hospital
LMU Munich
Marchioninistraße 15
81377 Munich
Germany

and

Medical Center FFB
Leonhardsplatz 2
82256 Fürstenfeldbruck
Germany

Chapter 1.3.

Dipl.-Ing. (FH) Margareta Santl
Dept. of Medicine III
LMU University Hospital
LMU Munich
Marchioninistraße 15
81377 Munich
Germany

Chapter 2.2.

Dr. rer. nat. Manfred Schmidt
Dept. of Radiation Oncology
University Hospital Erlangen
Universitätsstraße 27
91054 Erlangen
Germany

Chapters 1.1., 1.2.

Prof. Dr. med. Sabine Semrau
Dept. of Radiation Oncology
University Hospital Erlangen
Universitätsstraße 27
91054 Erlangen
Germany

Chapter 5.2.

Hana Dobšíçek Trefná
Biomedical Electromagnetics Group
Dept. Electrical Engineering
Chalmers University of Technology
412 96 Göteborg
Sweden

Chapter 2.3.

Dr. rer. nat. Tungte Wang
Dept. of Medicine III
LMU University Hospital
LMU Munich
Marchioninistraße 15
81377 Munich
Germany

Chapter 2.2.

Contents

1. Principles of Hyperthermia

1.1. Definition of Hyperthermia

The term *hyperthermia* has its origin in the Greek language and means *overheating or excessive heating*. To distinguish hyperthermia from other medical heat treatments, the following general definition of hyperthermia shall be used:

> Hyperthermia is a clinical treatment for malignant diseases, in which tumor tissue is exogenously heated to minimal temperatures of 40-41°C for a sufficiently long time.

This definition comprises four essential aspects that are important for clinical hyperthermia:

- The treatment aims at tumor remission or, at least, regression. Therefore, classical hyperthermia therapies must be clearly distinguished from other medical heating applications like muscle stimulation or other physical therapies.
- The heating is caused exogenously. It does not derive from physiological processes, but is generated by extracorporal or intracavitary/interstitial heating devices.
- The minimum effective temperature is generally assumed to be 40-41°C. At temperatures ≥42°C, cellular damage will continue to increase as temperatures increase due to the biological mechanisms associated with cellular heating, e.g. by coagulation of functional proteins. Even at temperatures as low as 40°C, cell destruction processes can be induced, and the effect of accompanying oncological standard therapies (radiotherapy and/or chemotherapy) can be intensified.
- The heating period must be sufficiently long. All desirable effects of hyperthermia only occur if the period of heating is long enough. The lower the temperature reached in the tumor tissue, the more time is usually needed for the desired therapeutic effect.

1.1.1. Different Temperature Regimes

It has been known for a long time that heating to high temperatures can be useful for tumor therapy. For many centuries, hot irons *("ferrum candens")* were used to cauterize smaller superficial tumors. Such a treatment offered several advantages in comparison to a purely surgical strategy: hyperthermia also heated a margin of surrounding normal tissue around the tumor where scattered tumor cells might have spread; in addition, hemorrhage was stopped, and the wound was sterilized by heat.

Furthermore, there were encouraging experiences with the therapeutic effects of heat at lower temperature levels (≤43°C). Sporadic case reports on patients with malignant diseases described marked tumor regressions or complete remissions after a history of strong fever [1].

Current therapeutic use of oncological heat treatments at different temperature levels:

■ Temperatures ≥50°C

In this temperature range, proteins coagulate rapidly, so that the tumor cells are destroyed after a comparably short heating time. High temperatures are achieved by the use of laser or electromagnetic radiation that is directly applied to the tumor tissue – mostly invasively. At these high temperature levels, it is very important to spare the surrounding normal tissues and organs, which are at risk. The invasive application and normal tissue tolerance usually limit the use of such high temperature methods. To distinguish these high temperature techniques from other heat treatments, they are designated as *thermoablation* [2, 3].

■ 41-45°C

Applications in this temperature range are mostly understood as *classical hyperthermia* in contrast to thermoablation. Here, a longer heating time is necessary to achieve tumor damage, but the potential for damage of the surrounding tissue is significantly reduced. The heating is often generated by electromagnetic radiation [4].

■ 40-43°C

This temperature range as a part of the classical hyperthermia temperature range is often distinguished from higher temperatures and it is referred to as *moderate hyperthermia*. Other biological mechanisms are important in this regime (☞ Chapter 1.3.). Usually hyperthermia in this temperature range is part of multimodal tumor treatments with the therapeutic aim to enhance a standard radio- and/or chemotherapy regimen [5-7]. The heating is often generated by electromagnetic radiation.

	Temperature range	Technique
Thermo-ablation	≥50°	laser, electrodes
Classical hyperthermia	41-45°C	electromagnetic radiation, ultrasound
Moderate hyperthermia	40-43°C	

1.1.2. Heating Techniques

On principle, all heating techniques that generate the required temperatures in the tumor tissue can be used for clinical hyperthermia. Sufficient energy deposition in the tumor is crucial, thereby sparing the surrounding tissue.

Electromagnetic radiation techniques are most frequently applied in hyperthermia treatments. Here the energy is delivered by antennas, electrodes or waveguides. Some systems use ultrasound for energy delivery. In thermoablation, lasers are often used. A new method is based on iron oxide nanoparticles that are put to the tumor cells. Using a fast oscillating magnetic field the nanoparticles are set in small oscillations that heat the tissue.

Further description is provided in Chapter 2.1.

1.1.3. References

1. Stoelben E, Koch M, Hanke S, et al. Spontaneous regression of hepatocellular carcinoma confirmed by surgical specimen: report of two cases and review of the literature. Langenbecks Arch Surg 1998;383:447-452.

2. Rehman J, Landman J, Lee D, et al. Needle-based ablation of renal parenchyma using microwave, cryoablation, impedance- and temperature-based monopolar and bipolar radiofrequency, and liquid and gel chemoablation: laboratory studies and review of the literature. J Endourol 2004;18:83-104.

3. Campos FG, Habr-Gama A, Kiss DR, et al. Management of the pelvic recurrence of rectal cancer with radiofrequency thermoablation: a case report and review of the literature. Int J Colorectal Dis 2005;20:62-66.

4. Vernon CC, Hand JW, Field SB, et al. Radiotherapy with or without hyperthermia in the treatment of superficial localized breast cancer: results from five randomized controlled trials. International Collaborative Hyperthermia Group. Int J Radiat Oncol Biol Phys 1996;35:731-744.

5. van der Zee J, Gonzalez Gonzalez D, van Rhoon GC, et al. Comparison of radiotherapy alone with radiotherapy plus hyperthermia in locally advanced pelvic tumours: a prospective, randomised, multicentre trial. Dutch Deep Hyperthermia Group. Lancet 2000;355:1119-1125.

6. Franckena M, Lutgens LC, Koper PC, Kleynen CE, van der Steen-Banasik EM, Jobsen JJ, et al. Radiotherapy and hyperthermia for treatment of primary locally advanced cervix cancer: results in 378 patients. Int J Radiat Oncol Biol Phys 2009;73:242-50.

7. Issels RD, Lindner LH, Verweij J, Wust P, Reichardt P, Schem BC, et al. Neo-adjuvant chemotherapy alone or with regional hyperthermia for localised high-risk soft-tissue sarcoma: a randomised phase 3 multicentre study. Lancet Oncol 2010;11:561-70.

1.2. Physical Basics and Hyperthermia Applications

Every physical method that leads to sufficient therapeutic heating of the tumor tissue and spares the surrounding normal tissue is applicable for clinical hyperthermia. However, the mostly applied hyperthermia techniques utilize electromagnetic radiation.

1.2.1. Electromagnetic Irradiation

Figure 1.1 shows the spectrum of electromagnetic radiation. Many different kinds of radiations are included as part of the electromagnetic radiation spectrum, e.g. radiowaves, light and X-rays.

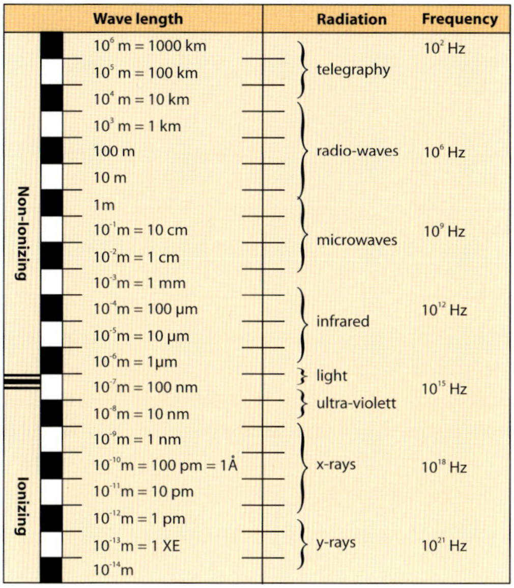

Figure 1.1: Spectrum of electromagnetic irradiation.

Every electromagnetic radiation consists of radiation particles called photons – the quantum particles of electromagnetic radiation. The only difference between the different forms of electromagnetic radiation is the energy of the photons that is given by:

$$E_{Photon} = h \cdot f = h \cdot \frac{c}{\lambda}$$

h = Planck constant, c = velocity of light, f = frequency, λ = wave length of the electromagnetic radiation.

All other basic physical properties are equal for such different radiation types as microwaves and X-rays. In hyperthermia, electromagnetic radiation in the range of radio- and microwaves is used.

The spectrum of electromagnetic radiation can be separated into two parts: ionizing and non-ionizing radiation (☞ Figure 1.1). In ionizing radiation, the radiation particles have enough energy to ionize atoms/molecules or to break up bindings of molecules, possibly leading to direct cell detriment if the DNA is hit. This requires energy in the range of several electron volts (eV). Thus, the border between ionizing and non-ionizing radiation lies in the region of ultraviolet radiation. In radiotherapy, the direct cell damaging ability of ionizing radiation is used to deactivate tumor cells. In hyperthermia, non-ionizing radiation is used with a particle energy that is not large enough to break up any bindings. The heating of the tissue is caused indirectly. However, if tissue is heated over a sufficient time at >41-42°C, proteins will coagulate and therefore cells will indirectly be damaged.

Table 1.1 compares the energetic aspects of hyperthermia to that of radiotherapy. Whereas in radiotherapy the energy of the single photons is larger by a factor of 10^{10}, in hyperthermia the total energy in one treatment fraction is larger by a factor of 10^4. This high total energy is necessary to raise the temperature measurably (an amount of 4.2 kJ is required to increase the temperature of one liter water by 1°C).

	Radiotherapy	Hyperthermia
Photon energy	1 MeV	1 µeV
Total energy per fraction	2 Gy × 5 kg = 10 J	278 W × 3600 s = 10^5 J

Table 1.1: A comparison of the energies in radiotherapy and hyperthermia.

Because electromagnetic radiation consists of quantum particles, the photons, a quantum theoretical treatment would be necessary for an exact description of the propagation and interaction of these photons with matter. In practice, with a very large number of photons, such a treatment would be, of course, too complex. Fortunately, there is an effective many particle theory that describes the phenomena of non-ionizing electromagnetic radiation very well: the classical electrodynamics. In this theory, the large number of propagating photons is described by an electromagnetic wave whose electric field strength is given in the special case of a plane wave propagating in z-direction in a homogeneous medium by:

$$\underline{E}(\underline{x}, t) = \underline{E}_0 \cdot \cos\left(\frac{360°}{\lambda} z - 360° \cdot f \cdot t + \phi_0\right)$$

$\underline{x}$ = the position in the three dimensional space, t = time, f = frequency, λ = wave length, $\underline{E}_0$ = amplitude (the maximum value) of the wave, ϕ_0 = the phase at time and position zero.

After a shift in z-direction by λ or a time shift by a period $T=1/f$ the wave has the same value again as is expected.

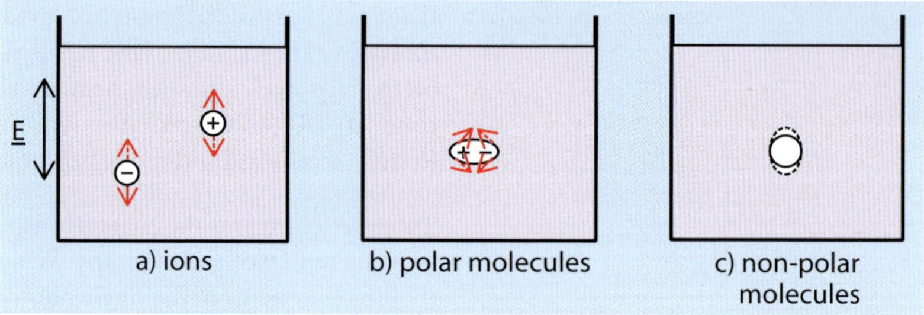

Figure 1.2: Schematic illustration of the absorption processes.

The wave term cos(...) is derived from the quantum theoretical wave function and E_0 is proportional to the square root of the number of photons. The argument of the cosine function is called the phase of the wave and gives the state of the wave (e.g. maximum, minimum or zero).

To this electric field, a magnetic field is also coupled by the Maxwell equations. However, because of its small influence to the tissue this magnetic field is negligible. So the effect of electromagnetic radiation is mainly described by the electric field strength $\underline{E}$ in the following.

1.2.2. Interaction of Non-Ionizing Electromagnetic Radiation with Matter

When non-ionizing electromagnetic radiation impacts on matter it can be reflected, transmitted (eventually with refraction), and partly absorbed. The possible absorption processes are illustrated in Figure 1.2.

The electric field influences the electric charges. If there are ions (a), then the oscillating electric field causes an oscillating movement of the ions, which hit the surrounding molecules. This leads to an increase of disorderly movement and consequently to heating. If there are polar molecules (b), the oscillating field causes a rotational movement of these molecules whereby they also hit the surrounding molecules. If there are only non-polar molecules or atoms (c), the oscillating field causes a deformation of the electron shell, which hits the surrounding molecules, resulting in heating.

From this consideration, it is clear that the heating is most effective in matter with freely moveable ions and least effective in solid matter with only non-polar molecules or atoms. These differences are given by the electric conductivity σ of the materials.

Absorption means an energy transfer from the electromagnetic wave to the matter and therefore leads to an attenuation of the electric field that, in homogeneous matter, is approximately described by an exponential attenuation. So, the above electric field comes to:

$$\underline{E}(\underline{x},t) = \underline{E}_0 \cdot \cos\left(\frac{360°}{\lambda} z - 360° \cdot f \cdot t + \phi_0\right) \cdot e^{-\frac{1}{2}\alpha \times d}$$

α = the absorption coefficient that gives the ability of energy absorption of the medium, d = depth in the matter.

Figure 1.3 shows the absorption coefficient of water as a function of the frequency of electromagnetic radiation. For soft tissue the shape of the graph is very similar. Three parts are distinguishable:

- In the range of light a minimum of absorption exists. Because there is a significant amount of water in the atmosphere, the eyes are adapted to this radiation.
- At higher frequencies the absorption coefficient decreases with increasing frequency. Therefore, photons with higher energy are more appropriate for deep-seated tumors in radiotherapy.
- At lower frequencies than light the situation is opposite. To achieve higher energy deposition in the depth, relative to the deposition at the surface, it is necessary to apply lower frequencies.

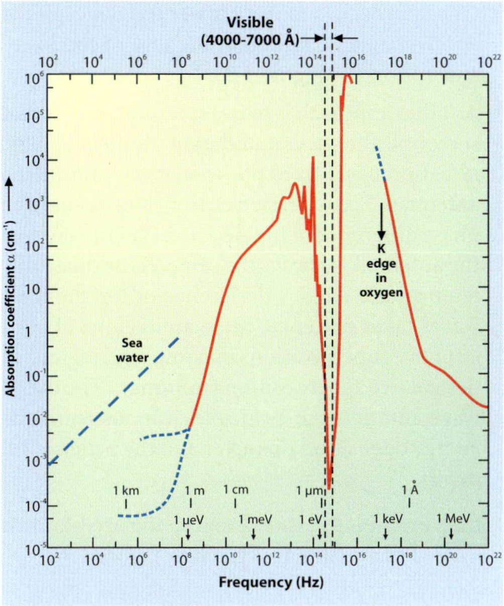

Figure 1.3: The absorption coefficient vs. the frequency for water [1].

The absorbed energy E_{abs}, at a point $\underline{x}$, is proportional to the number of photons ($\propto E^2$) that reach the point x integrated over the time:

$$E_{abs}(\underline{x}) \propto \int \left(E(\underline{x},t)\right)^2 dt$$

The proportional constant depends on the electric conductivity σ.

Another important quantity is the energy per time (= power) that is deposited in a small volume element or mass element. This quantity is called specific absorption rate (= SAR):

$$SAR(\underline{x},t) \propto \frac{E(\underline{x},t)^2}{\rho}$$

The SAR is also used in the field of harmful effects of mobile telephones and their emitting stations. It is comparable to the (energy) dose rate in radiotherapy. If it is large, a significant amount of energy is deposited in a small volume, which leads to a high heating. To achieve sufficient heating at a specific point a large electric field strength $\underline{E}$ is necessary at this point.

A further important point is the coupling of the antenna signal to the patient or tissue. Figure 1.4 shows the graph of the index of refraction n of water (similar to soft tissue) over the frequency.

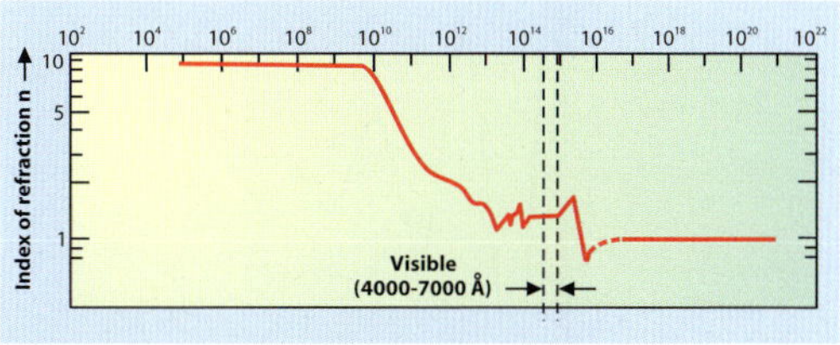

Figure 1.4: The index of refraction vs. the frequency for water [1].

The index of refraction for a medium gives the ratio of the propagation velocity of the radiation in the medium (water) and the velocity in vacuum (approximately equal to air). Because of $f = c/\lambda$ (f remains constant) n is also equal to the ratio of the wave length in the medium and in the vacuum :

$$n = \frac{c_{vacuum}}{c_{medium}} = \frac{f \cdot \lambda_{vacuum}}{f \cdot \lambda_{medium}} = \frac{\lambda_{vacuum}}{\lambda_{medium}}$$

In the range of radio- and microwave radiation, the refraction index has a value of about 10. This means that the wavelength is smaller in water than in air by this factor.

To have a good emission from the antenna in a medium; i.e. a good coupling to the medium, the size of the antenna must be adapted to the size of the wave length in the medium. Therefore, the antenna size should be in the order of magnitude of decimeter to irradiate tissue and not in the order of magnitude of meter, which would be necessary for a good emission in air. For the same reason it is also important that there is no air between the antenna and the patient to achieve a good coupling. In practice, this is accomplished using a flexible water bolus which adapts itself to the surface of the patient.

1.2.3. Practical Realizations

For a single source (e.g. antenna) of electromagnetic radiation in a typical frequency range from 400-1000 MHz, the electric field strength is already decreased to half after penetration into tissue by a depth of a few centimeters. This means that at a few centimeters depth the heating is clearly smaller than at the surface (☞ Figure 1.5).

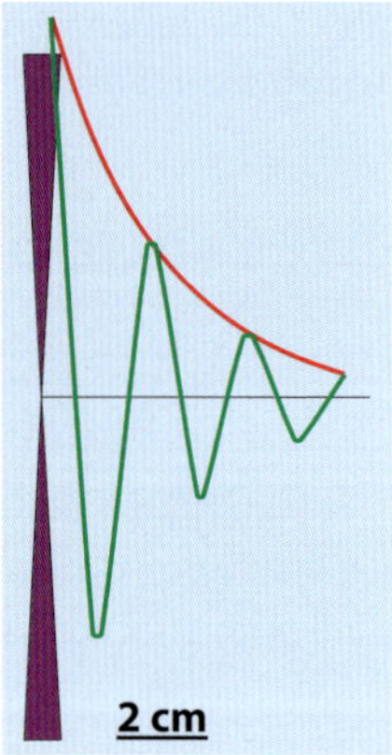

Figure 1.5: For explanations ☞ text.

However, if the surface is cooled by the water bolus, it is possible to homogeneously heat the tissue to a depth of a few centimeters (depending on the frequency of the radiation). Therefore, this application is applicable to superficial tumors like malignant melanomas or chest wall tumors. Of course, based on the size of the tumor, several antennas might be necessary to cover the whole region.

If a volume in larger depth has to be heated, it is possible to place several antennas at different depths (☞ Figure 1.6).

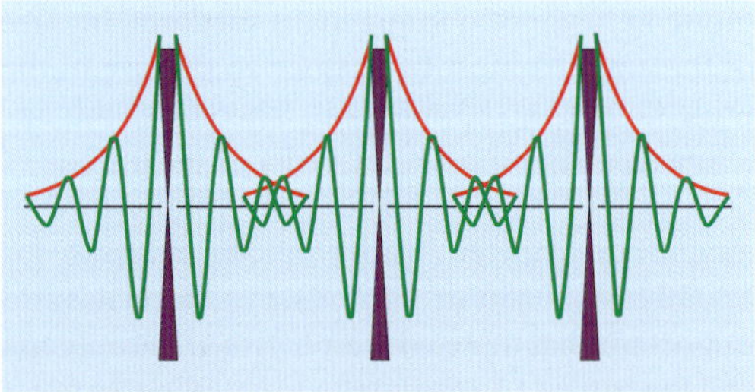

Figure 1.6: For explanations ☞ text.

Usually, surgical treatment is necessary to distribute the antennas in the whole tumor region. This is the application of interstitial hyperthermia, which is mainly used in combination with brachytherapy because the brachytherapy tubes can be used for insertion of the antennas.

The heating of deeper tumors or malignomas with a larger diameter without any surgical treatment is more difficult. Here, two techniques are applied to heat the tumor without harm to the surrounding tissue:

- One approach is to use a lower frequency of the electromagnetic radiation because of the lower absorption (☞ Figure 1.3).
- Another approach is to use several antennas that surround the patient and emit electromagnetic radiation using fixed phase relations among the antennas. Fixed phase relation means that the phase difference of the electromagnetic waves of the antennas is always the same. If the phase differences are fixed, interference of the different waves takes place; i.e. there are regions of constructive superposition (maxima) and regions of destructive superposition (minima). The use of wave interference principles can increase the energy deposition diameter and the penetration depth.

As an example of interference, the well-known double slit experiment is given in Figure 1.7a.

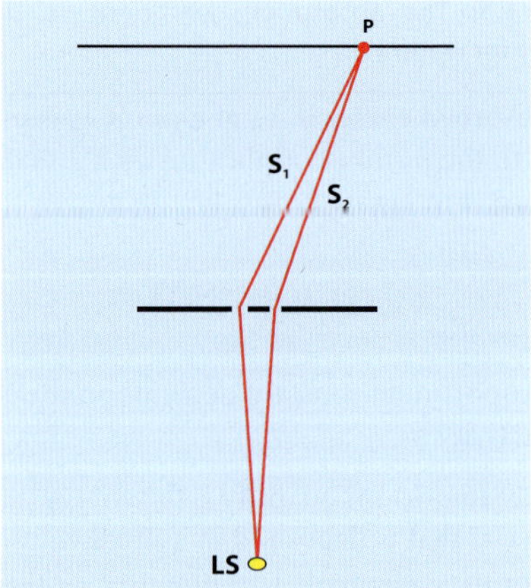

Figure 1.7a: Generation of interference pattern by two waves with fixed phase difference – the double slit experiment.

A light source (LS) shines through a double slit on a screen. The two slits can be seen as two "secondary" light sources with fixed phase relation because they are caused by the same light source. Therefore, interference takes place and generates an interference pattern on the screen – a change of maximum and minimum brightness. This pattern can be explained as follows:

From both slits a light wave arrives at point P on the screen. The distance between slit 1 and point P and the distance between slit 2 and the point P are s_1 and s_2, respectively. On the screen, brightness maxima always occur where the absolute difference

$$\Delta s = |s_1 - s_2|$$

is a multiple of the wave length, i.e.

$$\Delta s = n \cdot \lambda \quad n \in IN_0$$

because at these points both waves always have the same phase and so superpose constructively. If

$$\Delta s = n \cdot \lambda + \frac{\lambda}{2} \quad n \in IN_0$$

both waves always superpose with opposite phases that lead to extinction if the amplitudes are equal.

Figure 1.7b shows the analogue setting for a patient with two antennas on opposite sides.

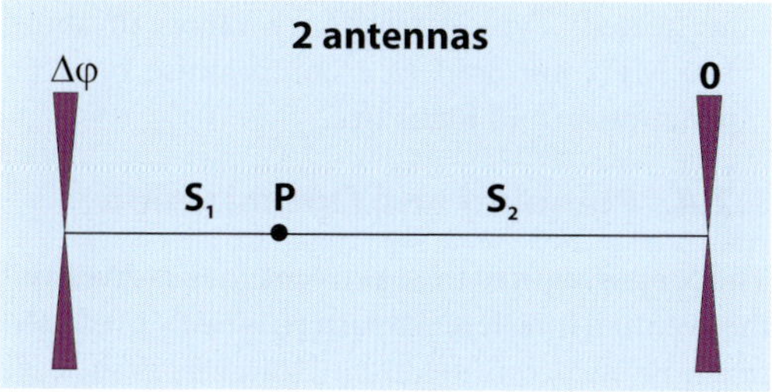

Figure 1.7b: Generation of interference pattern by two waves with fixed phase difference – setting for a patient with two antennas on opposite sides.

Here the superposition of the waves of both antennas also causes an interference pattern with maxima and minima, if the antennas have a fixed phase relation. If the antennas always send their signal with equal phase, the position of maxima and minima again depends on

$$\Delta s = |s_1 - s_2|$$

and a maximum will occur in the middle of the straight line between the antennas. As opposed to the double slit situation, here the phase relation between the sources can be freely chosen. So antenna 1 can start (t=0) with phase $\Delta\phi$, whereas antenna 2 starts with Phase 0. Then the two waves always have the fixed phase difference $\Delta\phi$. Then Δs is given by

$$\Delta s = \left| s_1 + \frac{\Delta\phi}{360°}\lambda - s_2 \right|$$

and the maximum is shifted by the half of $\lambda{\cdot}\Delta\phi\,/360°$ to the side of antenna 1. So it is possible to put the maximum to the tumor position.

The analogue is still valid if more than two antennas are used (e.g. four: ventral, dorsal, left and right of the patient). By an appropriate choice of the phase differences one can shift a maximum (called the focus) to the desired position.

Figure 1.8a shows the schematic setting of four antennas as it is typically used in applicators, Figure 1.8b shows the described focus steering perpendicular to the patient axis in a lamp phantom.

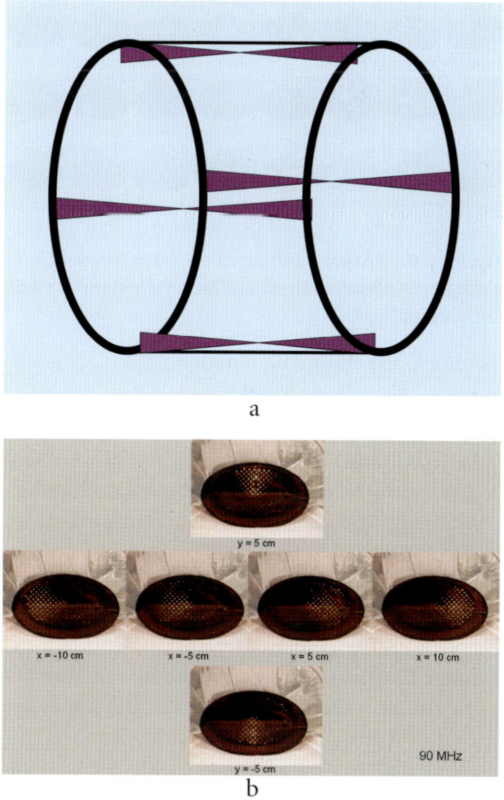

Figure1.8: Antenna setting of a 4 antennas applicator and steering of the focus perpendicular to the patient's axis (x-, y-coordinates).

In Figure 1.9a the arrangement of three rings consisting of four antennas is seen. With such a setting the focus can also be changed along the patient's axis (b).

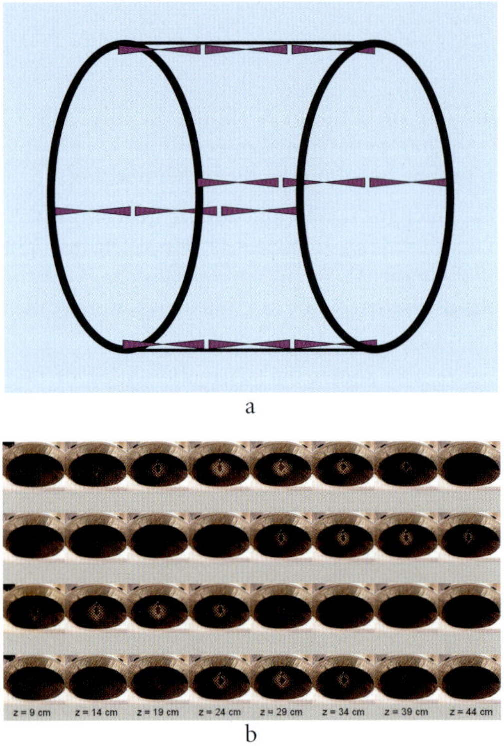

Figure 1.9: Antenna setting of a 3 × 4 antennas applicator and steering of the focus along the patient's axis (z-coordinate).

Three aspects should be noted:

- Because of the absorption of the radiation in an obese patient, the field strength is larger on the surface than at the focus position. This problem can usually be eliminated by bolus cooling. Additionally the antennas are constructed in an "H"-form to emit the energy on a larger area.
- Like in the double slit experiment, several maxima appear. In the typical four-antenna setting and homogeneous matter the maxima are arranged in the transversal plane like the dots of the five on a dice. If the patient is thicker or the central focus is shifted by a large distance, another maximum can occur inside the patient. This can lead to a hot spot in the healthy tissue.
- The term "focus" suggests that its size is small. Perpendicular to the antennas and transversal to the patient the size is in the magnitude of the distance between a maximum and a minimum; i.e., $\lambda/2 \propto 1/f$. Along the patient's axis the focus has the size in order of magnitude of the applicator-length.

There are three steering possibilities in such an antenna arrangement:

- By choosing appropriate phases, the focus can be shifted to the tumor.
- The amplitudes of the single waves can be changed. This mainly influences the patient's surface and can be used to avoid too much heating or not heating on the surface.
- The frequency of the electromagnetic radiation can be varied. A reduction of the frequency leads to:
  - a decrease of the absorption; i.e., the radiation penetrates the tissue better
  - an increase of the focus size in the transversal orientation

  That means that the frequency cannot be decreased to very low frequencies in order to have a better penetration because the focus would become too large and healthy tissue would also be heated. Typical frequency values of about 100 MHz are used as a compromise between penetration and focus size.

1.2.4. Planning and Optimization

The propagation of the electromagnetic waves and the eventual interference pattern is easily predicted in a homogeneous medium. However, in the case of electric inhomogeneous matter – like a patient – the situation is much more complex.

At every surface between different material reflections, refractions and phase shifts can lead to changes; e.g., the propagation or the interference pattern. Therefore it is very important to check the focus position using temperature probes in the inhomogeneous patient.

Theoretically, a calculation of the wave propagation and interference pattern is possible, if all the positions and electric properties of the different materials are known. For this, the surfaces, the volumes and the Maxwell equations are discretized and numerically solved. To lead to sufficiently exact results, knowledge of all the parameters, such as the electric properties and the location of the different tissues, is necessary – but is not always known.

The aim of hyperthermia is the heating of the tumor, while sparing the healthy tissue. Therefore, in addition to knowing the deposited energy (by the electric field) at every point, knowing the heat transport is very important, in order to estimate the temperature rise. The heat does not stay at the location where it is generated, but is carried off by heat conductivity and material transport (e.g. in vessels). These processes are theoretically calculable by the heat transport equation, but, again, an exact knowledge of the material properties, the locations and flow of the vessels are necessary and are usually not given.

For superficial and interstitial hyperthermia, planning and optimization is usually easy, because the tissue that surrounds the antennas can mostly be considered as homogeneous. However, special situations (e.g. a bone close to an antenna) can yield larger deviations between calculation and measurement and therefore, problems can occur during treatment.

In regional deep hyperthermia, where interference effects are used and energy is transmitted through different tissues, the above-mentioned aspects can lead to deviations between the planned and the actual temperature distribution. Therefore, temperature measurement is always very important during the treatment.

1.2.5. Harmful Effects of Non-Ionizing Radiation

When applying non-ionizing electromagnetic radiation it is important to consider potential harm and side effects for the patient and the staff. All possible effects can be distinguished as direct and indirect effects.

Direct effects

- Temporal varying electric and magnetic fields can cause charge movement and currents if there are moveable charged particles like ions. These currents can influence the nervous system and thereby lead to unpleasant stimulations and nervous disturbance. In the region of the heart the periodicity of the heart beat can also be disturbed. These electric current effects are only relevant at low frequencies (up to about 30 kHz), because at higher frequencies the charged particle cannot propagate sufficiently large distances in a half period of the oscillation.
- At higher frequencies the above-described heating effect dominates. This can lead to local burning of the tissue, but also – if large parts of the body are strongly heated – to disturbances of the circulatory system as it tries to cool the heated area.

Indirect effects

- By the electromagnetic radiation electric currents can be generated or charges can be separated in electric conducting material. The contact with such an object can cause a current in the body or burns if the object is heated by the induced currents.
- Electromagnetic radiation can also directly influence other electric or electronic devices and can interfere with their function. In the case of a cardiac pacemaker, this could have fatal consequences.

In spite of multiple speculations (as in the field of mobile telephones and their emitting stations), no further effects, including carcinogen effects, have been proven so far for non-ionizing radiation.

If hyperthermia is appropriately applied, none of the above-listed effects should occur to a patient. Only occasional low grade and mostly reversible burns are expected. It has to be ensured however that no, or at least no large, metal implants are located in the treatment region and that the patient has no active medical devices like a pacemaker in the region of influence of the electromagnetic radiation. If a large part of the body is heated, like in regional hyperthermia, the circulatory system (vital signs) should be controlled to avoid systemic overheating. This is especially important for patients with a weak circulatory system.

For the staff direct effects are not expected because the values of the SAR usually remain under the level and limits for such effects. To avoid indirect effects, one has to take care that there are no unintended and unchecked metal objects in the surrounding area . In the case of applicators with high power it is also important that the hyperthermia room is properly shielded. This is, however, not necessary because of possible effects to human beings, but rather because of the effects to other electric or electronic devices in the surrounding areas.

1.2.6. Further Heating Techniques

Heating by ultrasound

Here the energy is deposited by pressure waves instead of electromagnetic waves; i.e., by a change of high and low pressure in the tissue that generates periodic motion or displacements of the molecules within the tissue and produces heat from viscous friction losses. Many properties from the preceding sections are applicable to the ultrasound waves and are not repeated in this section. So in a homogeneous medium the pressure wave p in the special case of a plane wave propagating in z-direction in a homogeneous medium is again given as

$$p(\underline{x}, t) = p_0 \cdot \cos\left(\frac{360°}{\lambda} z - 360° \cdot f \cdot t + \phi_0\right)$$

The wave is emitted by an ultrasound transducer. The permanent oscillating pressure leads to a disorderly movement of the molecules resulting in heating. To heat and steer a large surface a moving transducer or a transducer array is necessary. Because the wavelength of ultrasound waves is some millimeters, interference effects cannot be applied to create a larger focus. To focus the heating, several waves from distinguished directions can be emitted by a curved transducer array. The use of this technique is limited by the small heating depth of some cm, the possible high reflections on boundaries and interfaces and that bone is heated stronger than soft tissue potentially causing pain.

Heating by infrared radiation

Infrared radiation can be used to heat superficial tumors, too. It is also a part of the electromagnetic spectrum. However, the wavelength is lower than that of microwaves, and the absorption is usually higher. A thin water layer between the source and the patient surface can absorb the parts with the highest absorption to get a more homogenous and deeper heating profile (water-filtered infrared-A hyperthermia). By this technique, therapeutic depths of some mm to 1 cm are possible.

Heating by nanoparticles

In this method of hyperthermia very small (superparamagnetic) iron oxide particles (size approx. 10 nm) are brought in the tumor. By a fast oscillating magnetic field these particles are forced to perform small oscillations whereby they interact with the surrounding molecules and cause disorderly movement leading to heating.

The challenges of this method are:

- Putting in and accumulating of the particles only in the tumor.
- The inhomogeneous heating caused by an inhomogeneous concentration of the nanoparticles.
- The nanoparticles remain in the patient and may cause side effects later.

So far, this technique is only used in clinical studies as an experimental method.

Heating in perfusion hyperthermia

Here, a chemotherapeutic agent or the blood circulates through the treatment region in the patient and a heating device outside the patient. In this device, the agent or the blood can be heated by any heating technique – like direct contact to a water bath or other heated objects. The heating of the tumor cells takes place by the contact with the agent or blood in the patient to reinforce the chemotherapy.

1.2.7. Heat Transport

After the energy deposition in the target volume using one of the methods described above, the temperature increases in the target region. However, the heat energy does not remain in this area but is carried off to the surrounding tissue. There are three different heat transport processes:

- *Exchange of warm and cold material – mainly by perfusion*
  In the target volume blood is also heated and flows into the surrounding tissue, whereas blood from colder regions reaches the heated volume and cools it down. At extended heating this perfusion process is increased by the circulatory system.
- *Heat conductivity by contact*
  If two objects of different temperatures are in contact, energy travels from the warmer to the colder one. In the patient, the heated target volume is always in contact with other tissue, so that heat transfer always takes place by heat conductivity.
- *Heat transport by electromagnetic radiation (e.g. infrared radiation)*
  Every object sends electromagnetic radiation to the surrounding area depending on its temperature (Stefan–Boltzmann law). This heat transport mechanism is very small at typical hyperthermia temperatures and only has a small range, making it negligible in hyperthermia.

The balance equation of these energy fluxes is called the heat transport equation.

An undesirable consequence of heat transport is that the tumor cannot be heated with a steep descent of temperature to the surrounding tissue. A further disadvantage is that the temperature distribution can be very inhomogeneous if there are larger blood vessels in or close to the target volume.

These effects can theoretically be considered by the heat transport equation but for that an exact knowledge of the material properties, the positions and flows of the vessels are necessary, but usually not given. Therefore, temperature measurement is very important during the treatment.

1.2.8. References

1. Jackson JD. Classical Electrodynamics, third edition 1999, John Wiley & Sons

1.3. Biological Rationale of Hyperthermia

1.3.1. Biological Rationale and Mode of Action of Hyperthermia

To understand the variety of biological effects of hyperthermia, it is mandatory to improve the effectiveness of this anti-cancer treatment. Nowadays, hyperthermia is part of multimodal treatment regimens consisting of surgery, radiotherapy, chemotherapy and, in future, most likely immune therapies. The studies on biological effects of hyperthermia encompass *in vitro* and *ex vivo* molecular cell biological and pre-clinical *in vivo* studies, complemented by monitoring of biological parameters of patients [1, 2]. The key biological modes of action of hyperthermia comprise direct cytotoxicity, chemosensitization, radiosensitization, modulation of the tumor micro-environment, and systemic effects that are strongly triggered by components of the immune system (summarized in [3, 4]).

But how can we assess the "biological dose" that is delivered by local heating? The specific absorption rate (SAR) is one measure of treatment delivery for electromagnetic hyperthermia methods as thermal dose parameter, but does not consider tissue-specific damage. However, in most tissue types, the cytotoxic time-dependent effects at 43°C are well understood and documented. Therefore, the Arrhenius equation-based cumulative equivalent minutes at 43°C (CEM43°C) value was introduced as a reference for the thermal dose, indicating the time required to produce a cytotoxic effect equivalent to the one found at at 43°C. In hyperthermia, CEM43°C is often referred to at 50 min ($CEM43T_{50}$) or at 90 min ($CEM43T_{90}$) and mainly represents the kinetics of cell killing by hyperthermia. Nevertheless, it has been a difficult task to define a thermal dose parameter that adequately predicts the plethora of biological effects caused by hyperthermia [5].

Following the results of research starting more than 50 years ago, a strict temperature-time relationship was noted for exponentially growing cells when exposed to heat shock above a threshold temperature [6]. The thermal energy dose for induction of cell death was found to be closely related to the amount of energy required for cellular protein denaturation, leading to the conclusion that the direct cytotoxic effect of hyperthermia itself is mainly based on denaturation and aggregation of unfolded proteins of nucleolic, cytoplasmatic or membrane proteins. These cytotoxic effects were in former times mostly related to proliferation and clonogenicity of the tumor cells. Meanwhile, it has become evident that several cell death forms can be induced by hyperthermia, such as apoptosis and necrosis [7].

Besides the direct effects of hyperthermia on tumor cells, tumor-selective effects at temperatures between 39°C and 43°C occur *in vivo*. One prominent example for this is the architecture of the vasculature in solid tumors, which is a chaotic one. This results in regions with hypoxia and low pH levels, which is not found in normal tissues with undisturbed conditions. Blood flow-related cooling during heating of tumors is therefore less than in normal tissue, meaning that the actual temperature rise obtained by the external heating devices can be higher than in the surrounding normal tissues. This renders tumor cells more sensitive to hyperthermia, especially in low-perfused areas. In addition, hyperthermia can also induce vascular damage and thereby indirectly tumor cell death. One has to note that small tumors require a higher SAR, as thermal conduction is the more prominent form of heat transfer [8].

A hyperthermia-induced increased metabolism of the tumor cells also increases anaerobic metabolism, resulting in acidosis and reduction of the cellular adenosine triphosphate (ATP) reservoir. Purine catabolites accumulate by ATP degradation together with formation of protons. ATP depletion is also one initiating step of necrotic cell death. Hyperthermia further increases cellular ceramide levels and membrane fluidity. All of the mentioned factors affect the viability and proliferation of tumor cells [9, 10].

A biological disadvantage intrinsically associated with hyperthermia is that one heat treatment can cause a transient resistance against a subsequent treatment (thermotolerance), because of the induction of stress proteins that, when located inside the cell, protect the cells from further damage. However, these compensatory mechanisms of heat shock proteins often fail to prevent cell death following exposure to more intense or prolonged heat shock and play important roles in tumor immunity, as demonstrated for the major stress-inducible heat shock protein Hsp70. Localization-dependent roles of Hsp70 have to be considered here [11].

As hyperthermia is clinically applied mainly in combination with chemo- and/or radiotherapy, its modes of action should be considered in these multimodal application settings.

1.3.2. Interaction of Hyperthermia and Chemotherapeutic Agents

Heat modifies the cytotoxicity of many chemotherapeutic agents and the thermal enhancement ratio (TER) is maximized at temperatures between 40.5 and 43.0°C (summarized in [12]). A hyperthermia-induced increase in blood perfusion in tumors improves tumor oxygenation and drug delivery in poorly vascularized tumor areas, thereby increasing local concentration of the chemotherapeutic agents. Besides physiological effects, synergy between heat and drugs may arise at the cellular level due to heat-induced damage to proteins or protein complexes involved in drug exclusion, in intracellular drug detoxification, and in repair of drug-induced DNA adducts.

Hyperthermia in combination with chemotherapy can lead to additive and supra-additive killing of tumor cells, especially in the case of alkylating agents, nitrosoureas, and some antibiotics. Also, cells with acquired drug resistance (often multifactorial) can again be made responsive to drugs by combining the drug treatment with heat, because heat acts at multiple levels to enhance drug toxicity. This has particularly been proven for cisplatin [13]. As one possible key mechanism is has been suggested that heat enhances the accumulation of platinum inside the cell and reduces its detoxification, leading to more DNA adducts. Table 1.2 shortly summarizes the diverse mechanisms that cause the cytotoxic properties of chemotherapeutic drugs to be affected by heat treatments.

1.3.3. Interaction of Hyperthermia and Ionizing Radiotherapy

Synergistic effects of radiotherapy and hyperthermia are mainly based on the complementary targets of these anti-cancer treatments. Tumor hypoxia represents a primary therapeutic concern for classical tumor therapies, because it reduces the

Drug	Cellular Target	Mechanism of heat to enhance cytotoxic properties of chemotherapeutic drugs
Alkylating agents	DNA strand breaks	Increased rate of alkylation
Cisplatin	Membranes and DNA	Increased drug uptake, increased DNA adducts and protein binding, increased cell death
Doxorubicin	Membranes and DNA	Increased drug uptake, increased drug half-life, increased oxygen radical production
Lonidamine	Mitochondria and enzymes	Decreased respiration
Mitomycin C	DNA	Increased radical production
Mitoxantrone	Membranes and DNA	Increased drug uptake, increased inhibition of topoisomerase II

Table 1.2: Modulation of cytotoxic properties of chemotherapeutics by hyperthermia.

effectiveness of radiotherapy and chemotherapeutic agents. Hypoxia may further reduce tumor sensitivity to ionizing radiation through indirect mechanisms that include proteomic and genomic changes. As already outlined in Chapter 1.3.1, hyperthermia leads to increased vascularization and enhanced vessel permeability, with an increase in oxygen pressure levels in the tumor and the tumor microenvironment that renders tumor tissue more radiosensitive.

Hyperthermia also weakens DNA damage repair enzymes such as BRCA2 [14] and thereby retards the repair of radiation-induced DNA damage [4]. Importantly, the synergy between radiation and heat is highest when applied closely together, i.e. within 4 hours [15]. Unfolded proteins and inactive protein aggregates are one central event by which heat sensitizes cells to radiation (summarized in [16]). When hyperthermia and radiotherapy are given sequentially, the synergy, often expressed as TER, is the highest. By increasing the time interval between first heat treatment and secondary radiation, the synergy is lost and the TER parallels the decline in protein aggregation. Indirect biochemical evidence further suggests that heat may exert its major effects on radiosensitivity via inhibiting the re-polymerization step in the repair of radiation-induced base damage (base excision repair), resulting in the formation of secondary toxic DNA double strand breaks [17].

Radiotherapy exerts its major effects in the G_2 phase, during mitosis, and in the G_1 phase of the cell cycle, while hyperthermia affects the S phase [6]. Taken together, hyperthermia is one of the most potent sensitizers for the action of ionizing radiation applied in radiotherapy [18] and has many complementary targets (summarized in Table 1.3).

	Hyperthermia	Radiotherapy
Oxygen pressure	low	high
pH value	acid tissue	basic tissue
Proteins	aggregation	oxidation
Cell cycle	S phase	G_2, M, G_1 phase
Cell death	modulation and amplification	induction

Table 1.3: Complementary targets of hyperthermia and radiotherapy.

1.3.4. Immune Modulation by Hyperthermia

Hyperthermia at 39-45°C has been demonstrated to modulate the innate and adaptive immune system [19, 20]. In dependence of the temperature, certain immunological processes are triggered. Starting with temperatures of 39°C, an increased infiltration and activation of immune cells in the tumor can be observed in pre-clinical model systems [21]. At higher temperatures, heat-induced cell death has certain characteristics of "immunogenic cell death (ICD)" [22]. This means that the dying and dead cells activate, rather than suppress, the immune system. In this scenario HSP70 is a major player. While inside the cell, it acts as chaperone and protects cells (thermotolerance), outside of the cell, e.g. when being released by heat-induced necrotic cells, it acts as a danger signal to activate dendritic cells (DCs) and deliver antigen to these key immune cells that bridge innate and adaptive immunity. Dendritic cells thus take up tumor antigens, present them with co-stimulation to $CD8^+$ T cells, and thereby induce cellular antitumor immunity by priming cytotoxic T lymphocytes [3]. Additionally, HSP70 can directly activate further cells of the innate immune system, such as natural killer cells [23]. Another prominent danger signal is the high mobility group box 1 (HMGB 1) protein. By combining hyperthermia with radiotherapy, increased amounts of HMGB1 are released [24]. Also, only after combination of heat and ionizing radiation, HSP70 is not only located at the tumor cell surface coupled to lipids, but also released into the extracellular space [25]. Furthermore, higher infiltration of DCs into tumors is observed [26]. Combination of hyperthermia and immune therapy with DCs was shown to increase the activity of cytotoxic T cells [27].

To summarize, hyperthermia, mostly in combination with radiotherapy, stimulates the priming phase of an immune response. However, tumors have developed escape mechanisms, e.g. by dampening the T cell responses. Here, the so-called immune checkpoint molecules (ICMs) are central. Under physiological conditions, ICMs assure that after initiation of a DC-mediated T-cell response, it is shut down later on to avoid autoimmunity [28]. Tumor cells use this mechanism to escape from immune surveillance. Recent research has

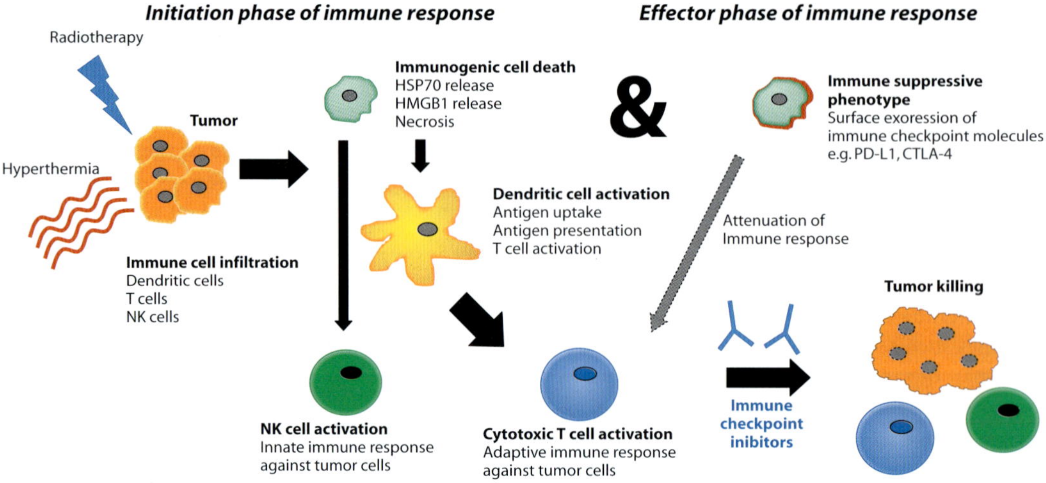

Figure 1.10: Hyperthermia in multimodal settings affects the initiation and effector phase of anti-tumor immune responses. CTLA-4: cytotoxic T lymphocyte antigen-4; HMGB1: high mobility group box 1 protein; HSP70: heat shock protein 70; NK: natural killer; PD-L1: programmed death-ligand.

proven that both radiotherapy and hyperthermia affect the expression of ICMs [29, 30]. Here, the form of heat application plays an additional role [31]. This suggests that in the future hyperthermia in multimodal tumor therapies should be combined with immune checkpoint inhibitors that target immune suppressive ICMs such as cytotoxic T lymphocyte antigen (CTLA-4) and programmed death-ligand 1 (PD-L1) or its receptor PD-1 [32]. The sequence of application of radiotherapy and hyperthermia seems to play a minor role when focusing on the immune phenotype of tumor cells [33]. In multimodal tumor treatments it should be beneficial to add distinct immune checkpoint inhibitors to the combination therapy of radio (chemo)therapy and hyperthermia to make use of the immune stimulatory properties of these treatments and to consecutively block the immune suppressive properties. In addition, thermal parameters have to be extendend that consider the manifold, dynamic and immunemodulatory properties of hyperthermia. Figure 1.10 summarizes the key effects of hyperthermia on the immune system in multimodal therapy settings.

1.3.5. References

1. Issels RD et al. Immune infiltrates in patients with localised high-risk soft tissue sarcoma treated with neo-adjuvant chemotherapy without or with regional hyperthermia: A translational research program of the EORTC 62961-ESHO 95 randomised clinical trial. Eur J Cancer 2021;158:123-132.

2. Sengedorj A et al. Interaction of radiotherapy and hyperthermia with the immune system: a Brief current overview. Current Stem Cell Reports 2022;8:129-138.

3. Hader M et al. Immune biological rationales for the design of combined radio- and immunotherapies. Cancer Immunol Immunother 2020;69(2):293-306.

4. Oei AL et al. Molecular and biological rationale of hyperthermia as radio- and chemosensitizer. Adv Drug Deliv Rev 2020;163-164:84-97.

5. van Rhoon GC. Is CEM43 still a relevant thermal dose parameter for hyperthermia treatment monitoring? Int J Hyperthermia 2016;32(1):50-62.

6. Bhuyan BK. Kinetics of cell kill by hyperthermia. Cancer Res 1979;39(6 Pt 2):2277-84.

7. Hader M et al. In vitro examinations of cell death induction and the immune phenotype of cancer cells following radiative-based hyperthermia with 915 MHz in combination with radiotherapy. Cells 2021;10(6):1436.

8. Adibzadeh F, MM Paulides, GC van Rhoon. SAR thresholds for electromagnetic exposure using functional thermal dose limits. Int J Hyperthermia 2018;. 34(8):1248-1254.

9. Busse M, P Vaupel. Accumulation of purine catabolites in solid tumors exposed to therapeutic hyperthermia. Experientia 1996;52(5):469-73.

10. Moulin M et al. Potential roles of membrane fluidity and ceramide in hyperthermia and alcohol stimulation of TRAIL apoptosis. Apoptosis 2007;12(9):1703-20.

11. Balogi Z et al. Hsp70 interactions with membrane lipids regulate cellular functions in health and disease. Prog Lipid Res 2019;74:18-30.

12. Issels RD. Hyperthermia adds to chemotherapy. Eur J Cancer 2008;44(17):2546-54.

13. Hettinga JV, AW Konings, HH Kampinga. Reduction of cellular cisplatin resistance by hyperthermia—a review. Int J Hyperthermia 1997;13(5):439-57.

14. Krawczyk PM et al. Mild hyperthermia inhibits homologous recombination, induces BRCA2 degradation, and sensitizes cancer cells to poly (ADP-ribose) polymerase-1 inhibition. Proc Natl Acad Sci USA 2011; 108(24):9851-6.

15. Elming PB et al. Hyperthermia: the optimal treatment to overcome radiation resistant hypoxia. Cancers (Basel), 2019;11(1):60.

16. Lepock JR. Role of nuclear protein denaturation and aggregation in thermal radiosensitization. Int J Hyperthermia 2004;20(2):115-30.

17. Iliakis G, W Wu, M Wang. DNA double strand break repair inhibition as a cause of heat radiosensitization: re-evaluation considering backup pathways of NHEJ. Int J Hyperthermia 2008;24(1):17-29.

18. Horsman MR, J Overgaard. Hyperthermia: a potent enhancer of radiotherapy. Clin Oncol (R Coll Radiol) 2007;19(6):418-26.

19. Repasky EA, SS Evans, MW Dewhirst. Temperature matters! And why it should matter to tumor immunologists. Cancer Immunol Res 2013;1(4):210-6.

20. Frey B et al. Old and new facts about hyperthermia-induced modulations of the immune system. Int J Hyperthermia 2012;28(6):528-42.

21. Chen Q et al. Photothermal Therapy Promotes Tumor Infiltration and Antitumor Activity of CAR T Cells. Adv Mater 2019;31(23):e1900192.

22. Galluzzi L et al. Consensus guidelines for the definition, detection and interpretation of immunogenic cell death. J Immunother Cancer 2020;8(1):e000337.

23. Multhoff G et al. The role of heat shock protein 70 (Hsp70) in radiation-induced immunomodulation. Cancer Lett 2015;368(2):179-84.

24. Schildkopf P et al. Application of hyperthermia in addition to ionizing irradiation fosters necrotic cell death and HMGB1 release of colorectal tumor cells. Biochem Biophys Res Commun 2010;391(1):1014-20.

25. Schildkopf P et al. Radiation combined with hyperthermia induces HSP70-dependent maturation of dendritic cells and release of pro-inflammatory cytokines by dendritic cells and macrophages. Radiother Oncol 2011; 101(1):109-15.

26. Werthmöller N et al. Combination of ionising radiation with hyperthermia increases the immunogenic potential of B16-F10 melanoma cells in vitro and in vivo. Int J Hyperthermia 2016;32(1):23-30.

27. Mukhopadhaya A et al. Localized hyperthermia combined with intratumoral dendritic cells induces systemic antitumor immunity. Cancer Res 2007;67(16):7798-806.

28. Pardoll DM. The blockade of immune checkpoints in cancer immunotherapy. Nat Rev Cancer 2012;12(4): 252-64.

29. Dovedi SJ et al. Acquired resistance to fractionated radiotherapy can be overcome by concurrent PD-L1 blockade. Cancer Res 2014;74(19):5458-68.

30. Stoll E et al. Detailed in vitro analyses of the impact of multimodal cancer therapy with hyperthermia and radiotherapy on the immune phenotype of human glioblastoma cells. Int J Hyperthermia 2022;39(1):796-805.

31. Hader M et al. Differences of the immune phenotype of breast cancer cells after ex vivo hyperthermia by warm-water or microwave radiation in a closed-loop system alone or in combination with radiotherapy. Cancers (Basel) 2020;12(5):1082.

32. Oei AL et al. Enhancing the abscopal effect of radiation and immune checkpoint inhibitor therapies with magnetic nanoparticle hyperthermia in a model of metastatic breast cancer. Int J Hyperthermia 2019;36(sup1): 47-63.

33. Sengedorj A et al. The effect of hyperthermia and radiotherapy sequence on cancer cell death and the immune phenotype of breast cancer cells. Cancers (Basel) 2022;14(9):2050.

2. Techniques, Clinical Use and Quality Assurance

2.1. Hyperthermia Treatment Techniques

2.1.1. Classical Techniques

Hyperthermia is a type of cancer treatment in which body tissue is exposed to moderately elevated temperatures to damage and kill cancer cells. Quality-assured hyperthermia is exclusively used in combination with established oncological standard treatments, such as chemo- and/or radiation therapy. Several classical methods of hyperthermia are in use, including local or superficial hyperthermia (LHT), interstitial hyperthermia (IHT), deep regional hyperthermia (RHT), and whole-body hyperthermia (WBHT). Targeted tumor temperatures for local and regional hyperthermia applications are 40-44°C and for whole body hyperthermia usually 41.5-42°C.

Superficial hyperthermia

Superficial hyperthermia (LHT) devices use various techniques that deliver energy to heat the tumor, e.g. microwaves, radiofrequency, and ultrasound. Generally, an external applicator is positioned directly over a localized tumor formation growing in the skin and/or the adjacent subcutaneous tissue, and energy is focused on the tumor to raise its temperature. In general, the penetration depth of therapeutic heat levels amounts to a few centimeters.

Typical clinical examples for the beneficial use of LHT in combination with radiotherapy are non-resectable chest wall recurrences of breast cancer after mastectomy [1, 2], local recurrences and in-transit metastases of malignant melanoma [1, 3], superficial soft tissue sarcoma [4], and locally advanced head and neck cancer [5, 6]. In randomized trials, additional LHT significantly improved local tumor control compared to irradiation alone [1-3, 5, 6].

Interstitial and endocavitary/intraluminal hyperthermia

Interstitial and endocavitary/intraluminal hyperthermia (IHT) methods may be used to treat tumors within or near body cavities, such as the esophagus or anal canal. Antennas are placed inside the cavity or interstitially direct to the tumor tissue to deliver energy and heat to the area directly. Interstitial hyperthermia is usually combined with interstitial brachytherapy. Within a short surgical procedure under general anesthesia, several afterloading tubes are inserted into the malignant tissue for brachytherapy. Before and/or after irradiation, dedicated heat sources (e.g. antennas) are placed within the brachytherapy tubes to additionally heat the target lesion. In clinical trials, additional IHT has been shown to improve relevant clinical endpoints, e.g. overall survival and/or local recurrence rates of patients with bladder cancer [7] and glioblastoma multiforme [8].

Interstitial and intraluminal hyperthermia has been also used in combination with prostate brachytherapy [9] for adenocarcinoma of the prostate gland or in the additive hyperthermic treatment of anal [10], and esophageal cancer [11], as part of a multimodal treatment schedule containing radiotherapy and/or chemotherapy.

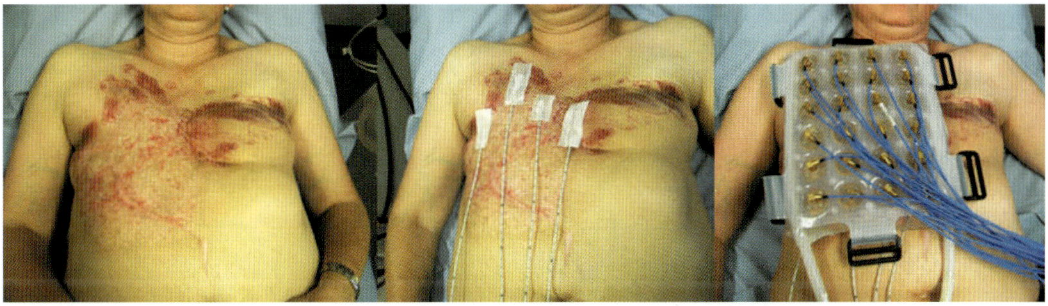

Figure 2.1: Left: Female Patient with an extended inflammatory breast cancer chest wall recurrence. Middle: Superficial thermometry catheters. Right: 24-channel superficial hyperthermia applicator.

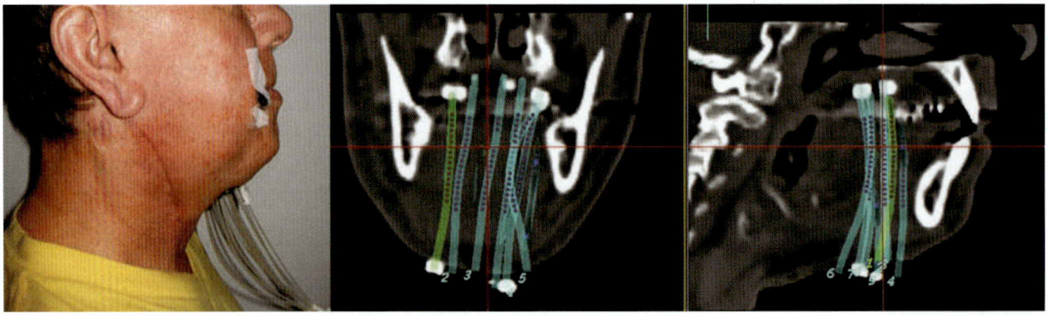

Figure 2.2: Male patient with a recurrent squamous cell cancer of the floor of mouth. Implanted brachytherapy catheters for small volume pulsed-dose-rate salvage reirradiation combined with concurrent chemotherapy and interstitial hyperthermia.

Deep Regional Hyperthermia

For locally advanced carcinomas of the abdomen, pelvis, and extremities, deep regional hyperthermia (RHT) is recommended. External applicators are positioned around the body cavity or organ to be treated, and microwave or radiofrequency energy is focused on the area to raise its temperature. The clinical efficacy of RHT had been proven in randomized trials in locally advanced cervical carcinoma [12, 13], rectal cancer [14], and soft tissue sarcoma [15, 16]. Further indications for the additional use of RHT in combination with radiochemotherapy, radiotherapy, and chemotherapy are locally recurrent rectal [17, 18], bladder [19, 20], prostate [21], anal [10, 22], pancreatic [23, 24] and gastric cancer [25].

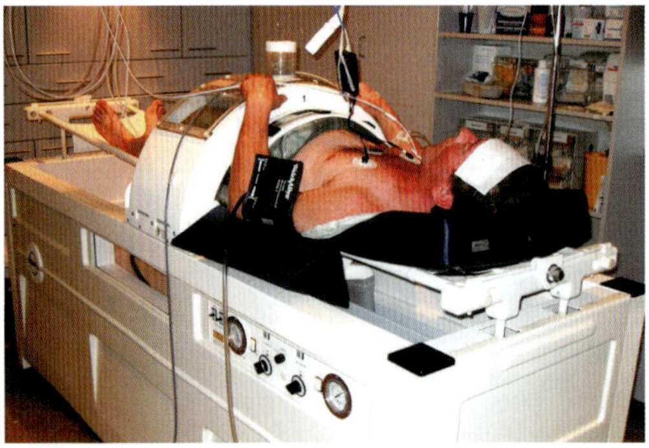

Figure 2.3: Male patient with anal cancer receiving deep regional hyperthermia during a series of standard chemoradiation.

Another regional hyperthermia approach includes perfusion techniques [26] that can be used to treat cancers in the arms and legs, such as melanomas, or cancer in some organs, such as the liver or lung. In one type of perfusion procedure, some of the patient's blood is removed, heated, and then perfused back into the limb or organ. Anticancer drugs are commonly given during this treatment. Continuous hyperthermic peritoneal perfusion (HIPEC) is a technique used to treat cancers within the peritoneal cavity, including primary peritoneal mesothelioma, gastric and ovarian cancer [27]. During surgery, heated anticancer drugs flow from a warming device through the peritoneal cavity. The peritoneal cavity temperature reaches 41-42°C [28].

Whole-body hyperthermia

Whole-body hyperthermia (WBHT) is used to treat metastatic cancer that has spread throughout the body. Several techniques that raise the body temperature to 41.5-42°C, including the use of thermal chambers (similar to large incubators) or hot water blankets can accomplish this. The aim of additional hyperthermia combined with systemic chemotherapy was to enhance its antitumor effect, and WBHT was predominantly used in patients with incurable metastasized malignancies who developed progressive disease after first or second line systemic treatment. Some phase II trials proved the feasibility of WBHT with chemotherapy for metastasized rectal, prostate and ovarian cancer, but an explicit benefit for the additional use of WBHT could not be shown because of the lack of randomized trials [29, 30]. In evidence-based medicine, WBHT does not currently receive much attention.

2.1.2. Recent Developments

Non-invasive thermometry with MRI scanners

The combination of deep regional hyperthermia systems combined with non-invasive MRI-thermometry has been established worldwide in some major oncological departments during the past 15 years. Controlling the effect of hyperthermia during patient treatment is essential for quality-controlled therapy. However, standard invasive temperature measurements of the body tissue and in natural orifices monitor only representative tissue points. The addition of thermal mapping (scanning the temperature probes along the catheter tracks) provides much more information about the temperature in the tumor and normal tissue. Using the combination of a deep regional hyperthermia system with an MRI-scanner, the physician obtains three-dimensional information about temperature and perfusion during the hyperthermia. After short MR measuring sequences, the operator transfers the image data to a hyperthermia planning workstation, and, within less than two minutes, color-coded temperature distribution images covering the whole region of interest are available for review, allowing for the immediate optimization of the treatment parameters. With the introduction of non-invasive MR-thermometry techniques, RHT treatment quality is expected to further improve effective heating of tumors and avoid painful hot spots in the surrounding normal tissue [31, 32].

Magnetic hyperthermia

A stable bio-inert colloid of coated iron oxide nanoparticles dispersed in water (Magnetic Fluid) is applied interstitially into a target region containing the tumor or is immobilized in a biodegradable matrix which is placed onto the resection cavity wall during tumor resection (intra-cavitary "NanoPaste"). This magnetic fluid is subsequently heated by an external AC magnetic field applicator system ("NanoActivator"). Based on conventional post-application CT-scans, a temperature simulation software calculates the specific absorption rate (SAR) in W/g tissue for a certain magnetic field strength. Using this energy term, the same software is able to calculate the temperature gradients within full CT image resolution after solving the bioheat transfer equation (BTE). The temperature cannot be predicted precisely as the most unknown parameter in the BTE is the tumor perfusion, which can vary in particular during heating based on thermoregulation and after thermal damage of the tumor vascular system. Thus, a minimal invasive fluorooptical thermometry is part of the so-called

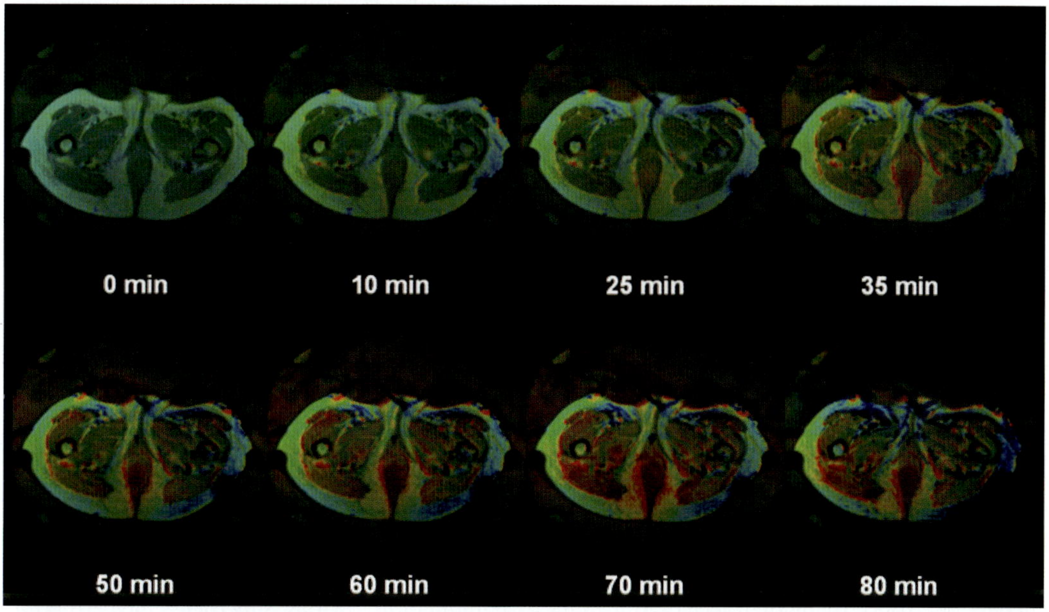

Figure 2.4: MR-thermometry during a deep regional hyperthermia treatment for a female patient with anal cancer. The increase in red color shows the temperature increase in the target region.

NanoTherm Therapy System (NTTS), which allows continuous intratumoral temperature measurements during the magnetic field application. This technique using magnetic nanoparticles falls under the regional hyperthermia category as regions of the body can be easily selected to be heated, even for tumors that are positioned deeper inside. Whereas the nanoparticles are minimally invasively applied, forming stable deposits within the target tissue, all subsequent magnetic field applications (activation of the particles) are contactless to the patient. The nanoparticles are applied once. The magnetic field application (thermotherapy) is repeated twice a week, 6 times total, 60min each. The method is based on a defined and very efficient transfer of power onto magnetic nanoparticles in an alternate magnetic field that is determined by the type of particles, frequency and magnetic field strength, which results in local generation of heat [33]. Depending on the equilibrium temperature set in the tumor tissue, this heat may either destroy the tumor cells directly (thermoablation) or result in a synergic reinforcement of radiation efficacy (hyperthermia). Magnetic hyperthermia has been tested in several clinical trials for various tumors [34]; e.g., in the treatment of glioblastoma multiforme [35, 36], prostate cancer [37, 38] and locally recurrent tumors [39]. Intracavitary thermotherapy combined with radiotherapy can induce a prominent inflammatory reaction around the resection cavity which might trigger potent antitumor immune responses possibly leading to long-term stabilization of recurrent GBM patients [40]. Histological analysis and flow cytometry of tissue acquired during removal of the nanoparticles showed increased infiltration of CD8+ T cells, CD4+ T cells and CD63+ macrophages in areas containing large numbers of nanoparticles, indicating that an immune response had been triggered. The combination of fluorescence-guided resection using 5-aminolevulinic acid (5-ALA) and intracavitary thermotherapy provides a novel and promising treatment option for improving local tumor control in recurrent high-grade gliomas, but further refinements of the treatment protocol are needed to decrease major side effects [41]. Repeated cycles of thermotherapy can be administered without additional surgery, and the treatment has the potential to synergize with radiotherapy or chemotherapy. A prospective phase II trial examined the feasibility of magnetic hyperthermia in 59 patients with recurrent glioblastoma [42]. Possible improvements in survival were found, although some patients experienced adverse effects, such as seizures during treatment or worsening of motor disturbances after treatment. Intracavitary magnetic hyperthermia seems to induce a potent inflammatory response, and as glioblastomas are known to be immunologically 'cold' tumors, this therapy might help improve the immune response and/or the efficacy of immune therapies [43, 44].

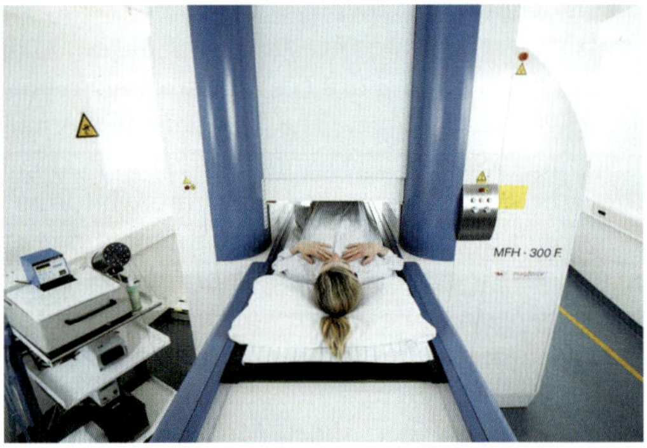

Figure 2.5: Patient receiving Magnetic Fluid Hyperthermia.

Thermosensitive liposomes

Specifically designed liposomes which are stable at physiologic temperatures of 37-38°C and which release their content at temperatures of about 40-43°C have been developed to enable tumor-selective drug delivery in combination with regional hyperthermia. Typically, these liposomes lack cholesterol and are composed of palmitoyllecithins with a phase transition temperature (Tm) of 41.5°C. Heating thermosensitive liposomes (TSL) above Tm leads to an increase in lipid hydrocarbon chain mobility, rendering the membrane leaky for small molecules. By the addition of lysolecithins, these liposomes show an ultrafast drug release upon heating, with a total release of the encapsulated drug within 20 seconds [45]. Doxorubicin is the most frequently used anticancer drug in liposomes, as it can be actively loaded by a pH gradient method with a more than 95% loading efficiency. Lysolecithins containing TSL have shown superior activity, in an animal tumor model, over conventional TSL, and are under clinical investigation for chest wall recurrences of breast cancer in combination with superficial hyperthermia (ThermoDOX®, Phase I/II) and for hepatocellular carcinoma in combination with radiofrequency ablation [46]. The intravascular drug release properties seem to be a key issue for these liposomes. An alternative approach is based on the novel lipid class of phosphatidyloligoglycerols, which leads to TSL with prolonged plasma circulation time and comparable fast drug release properties [47, 48].

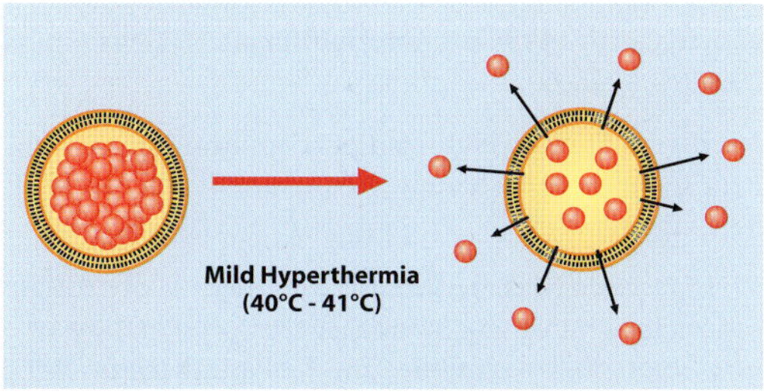

Figure 2.6: Thermosensitive liposomes releasing chemotherapy in combination with mild hyperthermia.

2.1.3. References

1. Jones EL, Oleson JR, Prosnitz LR, et al. Randomized trial of hyperthermia and radiation for superficial tumors. J Clin Oncol 2005;23:3079-3085.

2. Vernon CC, Hand JW, Field SB, et al. Radiotherapy with or without hyperthermia in the treatment of superficial localized breast cancer: results from five randomized controlled trials. International Collaborative Hyperthermia Group. Int J Radiat Oncol Biol Phys 1996; 35:731-744.

3. Overgaard J, Gonzalez Gonzalez D, Hulshof MC, et al. Randomised trial of hyperthermia as adjuvant to radiotherapy for recurrent or metastatic malignant melanoma. European Society for Hyperthermic Oncology. Lancet 1995;345:540-543.

4. Datta NR, Bose AK, Kapoor HK, et al. Head and neck cancers: results of thermoradiotherapy versus radiotherapy. Int J Hyperthermia 1990;6:479-486.

5. Datta NR et al., Head and neck cancers: results of thermoradiotherapy versus radiotherapy. Int J Hyperthermia 1990;6(3):479-86.

6. Valdagni R, M Amichetti. Report of long-term follow-up in a randomized trial comparing radiation therapy and radiation therapy plus hyperthermia to metastatic lymph nodes in stage IV head and neck patients. Int J Radiat Oncol Biol Phys 1994;28(1):163-9.

7. Colombo R et al. Multicentric study comparing intravesical chemotherapy alone and with local microwave hyperthermia for prophylaxis of recurrence of superficial transitional cell carcinoma. J Clin Oncol 2003; 21(23):4270-6.

8. Sneed PK et al. Survival benefit of hyperthermia in a prospective randomized trial of brachytherapy boost +/- hyperthermia for glioblastoma multiforme. Int J Radiat Oncol Biol Phys 1998;40(2):287-95.

9. Van Vulpen M et al. Radiotherapy and hyperthermia in the treatment of patients with locally advanced prostate cancer: preliminary results. BJU Int 2004;93(1):36-41.

10. Kouloulias V et al. Chemoradiotherapy combined with intracavitary hyperthermia for anal cancer: feasibility and long-term results from a phase II randomized trial. Am J Clin Oncol 2005;28(1):91-9.

11. Qi C, DJ Li. Thermometric analysis of intra-cavitary hyperthermia for esophageal cancer. Int J Hyperthermia 1999;15(5):399-407.

12. Franckena M et al. Radiotherapy and hyperthermia for treatment of primary locally advanced cervix cancer: results in 378 patients. Int J Radiat Oncol Biol Phys 2009; 73(1):242-50.

13. van der Zee J et al. Comparison of radiotherapy alone with radiotherapy plus hyperthermia in locally advanced pelvic tumours: a prospective, randomised, multicentre trial. Dutch Deep Hyperthermia Group. Lancet 2000; 355(9210):1119-25.

14. De Haas-Kock DF et al. Concomitant hyperthermia and radiation therapy for treating locally advanced rectal cancer. Cochrane Database Syst Rev 2009(3):CD006269.

15. Issels RD et al. Effect of neoadjuvant chemotherapy plus regional hyperthermia on long-term outcomes among patients with localized high-risk soft tissue sarcoma: The EORTC 62961-ESHO 95 randomized clinical trial. JAMA Oncol 2018;4(4):483-492.

16. Issels RD et al. Neo-adjuvant chemotherapy alone or with regional hyperthermia for localised high-risk soft-tissue sarcoma: a randomised phase 3 multicentre study. Lancet Oncol 2010;11(6):561-70.

17. Juffermans JH et al. Reirradiation and hyperthermia in rectal carcinoma: a retrospective study on palliative effect. Cancer 2003;98(8):1759-66.

18. Ott OJ et al. Neoadjuvant chemoradiation combined with regional hyperthermia in locally advanced or recurrent rectal cancer. Cancers (Basel) 2021;13(6).

19. Merten R et al. Long-term experience of chemoradiotherapy combined with deep regional hyperthermia for organ preservation in high-risk bladder cancer (Ta, Tis, T1, T2). Oncologist 2019;24(12):e1341-e1350.

20. Ott OJ et al. Radiochemotherapy for bladder cancer. Clin Oncol (R Coll Radiol) 2009;21(7):557-65.

21. Tilly W et al. Regional hyperthermia in conjunction with definitive radiotherapy against recurrent or locally

advanced prostate cancer T3 pN0 M0. Strahlenther Onkol 2005;181(1):35-41.

22. Ott OJ et al. Chemoradiotherapy with and without deep regional hyperthermia for squamous cell carcinoma of the anus. Strahlenther Onkol 2019;195(7):607-614.

23. Issels RD et al. Regional hyperthermia with cisplatin added to gemcitabine versus gemcitabine in patients with resected pancreatic ductal adenocarcinoma: The HEAT randomised clinical trial. Eur J Cancer 2023;181: 155-165.

24. Schlemmer M et al. [Principles, technology and indication of hyperthermia and part body hyperthermia]. Radiologe 2004;44(4):301-9.

25. Mochiki E et al. Feasibility study of postoperative intraperitoneal hyperthermochemotherapy by radiofrequency capacitive heating system for advanced gastric cancer with peritoneal seeding. Int J Hyperthermia 2007; 23(6):493-500.

26. Cornett WR et al. Randomized multicenter trial of hyperthermic isolated limb perfusion with melphalan alone compared with melphalan plus tumor necrosis factor: American College of Surgeons Oncology Group Trial Z0020. J Clin Oncol 2006;24(25):4196-201.

27. van Rhoon GC, M Franckena, TLM Ten Hagen. A moderate thermal dose is sufficient for effective free and TSL based thermochemotherapy. Adv Drug Deliv Rev 2020;163-164:145-156.

28. Verwaal VJ et al. 8-year follow-up of randomized trial: cytoreduction and hyperthermic intraperitoneal chemotherapy versus systemic chemotherapy in patients with peritoneal carcinomatosis of colorectal cancer. Ann Surg Oncol 2008;15(9):2426-32.

29. Dawczak-Debicka A et al. Complementary and alternative therapies in oncology. Int J Environ Res Public Health 2022;19(9):5071.

30. Hildebrandt B et al. Current status of radiant whole-body hyperthermia at temperatures >41.5 degrees C and practical guidelines for the treatment of adults. The German 'Interdisciplinary Working Group on Hyperthermia'. Int J Hyperthermia 2005;21(2):169-83.

31. Feddersen TV et al. Multi-echo gradient echo pulse sequences: which is best for PRFS MR thermometry guided hyperthermia? Int J Hyperthermia 2023;40(1): 2184399.

32. Gellermann J et al. Noninvasive magnetic resonance thermography of soft tissue sarcomas during regional hyperthermia: correlation with response and direct thermometry. Cancer 2006;107(6):1373-82.

33. Jordan A et al. Inductive heating of ferrimagnetic particles and magnetic fluids: physical evaluation of their potential for hyperthermia. Int J Hyperthermia 1993; 9(1):51-68.

34. Thiesen B, A Jordan. Clinical applications of magnetic nanoparticles for hyperthermia. Int J Hyperthermia 2008;24(6):467-74.

35. Maier-Hauff K et al. Intracranial thermotherapy using magnetic nanoparticles combined with external beam radiotherapy: results of a feasibility study on patients with glioblastoma multiforme. J Neurooncol 2007;81(1):53-60.

36. Rivera D et al. Neurosurgical applications of magnetic hyperthermia therapy. Neurosurg Clin N Am 2023; 34(2):269-283.

37. Johannsen M et al. Clinical hyperthermia of prostate cancer using magnetic nanoparticles: presentation of a new interstitial technique. Int J Hyperthermia 2005; 21(7):637-47.

38. Johannsen M et al. Magnetic nanoparticle hyperthermia for prostate cancer. Int J Hyperthermia 2010; 26(8):790-5.

39. Wust P et al. Magnetic nanoparticles for interstitial thermotherapy—feasibility, tolerance and achieved temperatures. Int J Hyperthermia 2006;22(8):673-85.

40. Grauer O et al. Combined intracavitary thermotherapy with iron oxide nanoparticles and radiotherapy as local treatment modality in recurrent glioblastoma patients. J Neurooncol 2019;141(1):83-94.

41. Schwake M et al. Combined fluorescence-guided resection and intracavitary thermotherapy with superparamagnetic iron-oxide nanoparticles for recurrent high-grade glioma: Case series with emphasis on complication management. Cancers (Basel) 2022;14(3):541.

42. Maier-Hauff K et al. Efficacy and safety of intratumoral thermotherapy using magnetic iron-oxide nanoparticles combined with external beam radiotherapy on patients with recurrent glioblastoma multiforme. J Neurooncol 2011;103(2):317-24.

43. Brown NF et al. Harnessing the immune system in glioblastoma. Br J Cancer 2018;119(10):1171-1181.

44. van Solinge TS et al. Advances in local therapy for glioblastoma - taking the fight to the tumour. Nat Rev Neurol 2022;18(4):221-36.

45. Needham D et al. A new temperature-sensitive liposome for use with mild hyperthermia: characterization and testing in a human tumor xenograft model. Cancer Res 2000;60(5):1197-201.

46. Borys N, MW Dewhirst. Drug development of lysothermosensitive liposomal doxorubicin: Combining hyperthermia and thermosensitive drug delivery. Adv Drug Deliv Rev 2021;178:113985.

47. Lindner LH et al. Novel temperature-sensitive liposomes with prolonged circulation time. Clin Cancer Res 2004;10(6):2168-78.

48. Zimmermann K et al. A pilot trial of doxorubicin containing phosphatidyldiglycerol based thermosensitive liposomes in spontaneous feline soft tissue sarcoma. Int J Hyperthermia 2017;33(2):178-190.

2.2. Practical Recommendations

The practical recommendations for hyperthermia procedures are defined according to the European Society for Hyperthermic Oncology (ESHO) Quality Assurance Guidelines for regional hyperthermia treatment [1-6] and our experience in the treatment of patients with deep-seated and superficial tumors. Deep-seated tumors are located under the skin fascia, especially tumors which are located in retroperitoneal cavity (rectal and pancreatic carcinomas, soft tissue sarcomas). Superficial tumors grow on the tissue surface without growing into deeper layers or adjacent organs such as recurrent breast cancer after ablation or superficial soft tissue sarcomas. The outcome of hyperthermia-combined therapies relies strongly on the quality of the applied heat treatment and consequently the achieved tumor temperature [4-6]. The primary objective of quality assurance guidelines for regional hyperthermia (RHT) is to guarantee the optimal propagation of the electromagnetic waves to focus the energy on the target lesion with simultaneous protection of the surrounding healthy tissue to be able to produce therapeutic temperatures in the tumor. A secondary objective is the improvement of the patient's comfort.

Retroperitoneal and pelvic tumors are deep-seated and highly perfused, which makes them difficult to heat. In addition, if their location is in the upper abdomen (e.g. pancreatic cancer), it is difficult to position the applicator correctly on the center of the tumor lesion, at least in small patients. The devices most often employed for heating of deep-seated malignancies are concentric arrays of high frequency electromagnetic applicators such as Sigma 60/Sigma-Eye Applicators (Pyrexar Medical Corporation, Salt Lake city, Utah, USA) and ALBA Systems (MED-LOGIX SRL, Rome, Italy). The radiative Sigma-Eye applicator contains 24 adjustable antennas providing three-dimensional steering in radial and longitudinal direction.

Figure 2.7 shows the BSD-2000 deep regional hyperthermia system with both applicators (SIGMA-Eye and SIGMA-60) including the sche-

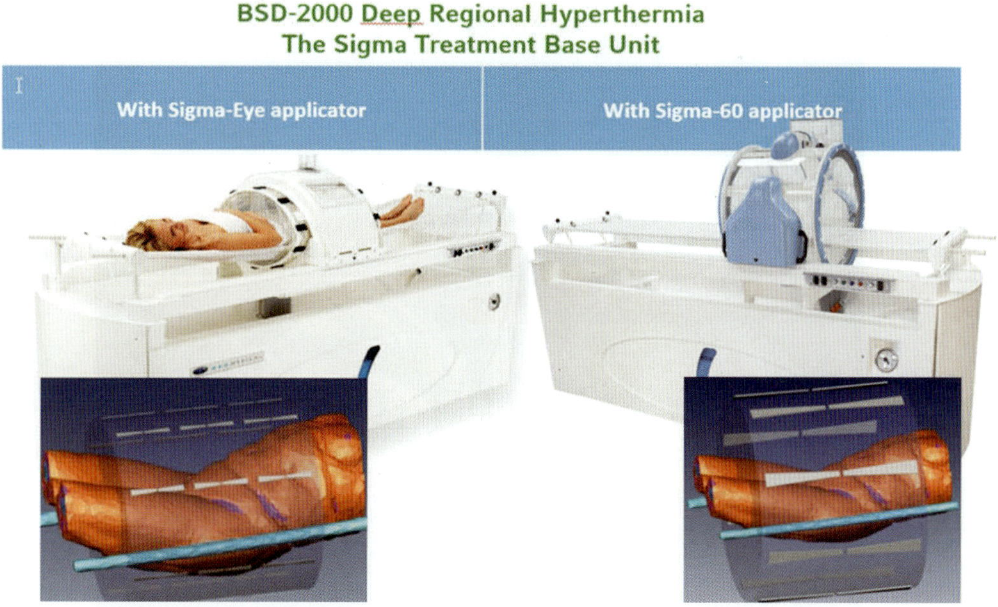

Figure 2.7: The BSD regional hyperthermia System with both Applicators Sigma-Eye and Sigma-60 with the schematic representation of the antennas in both applicators (Photo provided by Company Sennewald Medizintechnik, Munich, Germany).

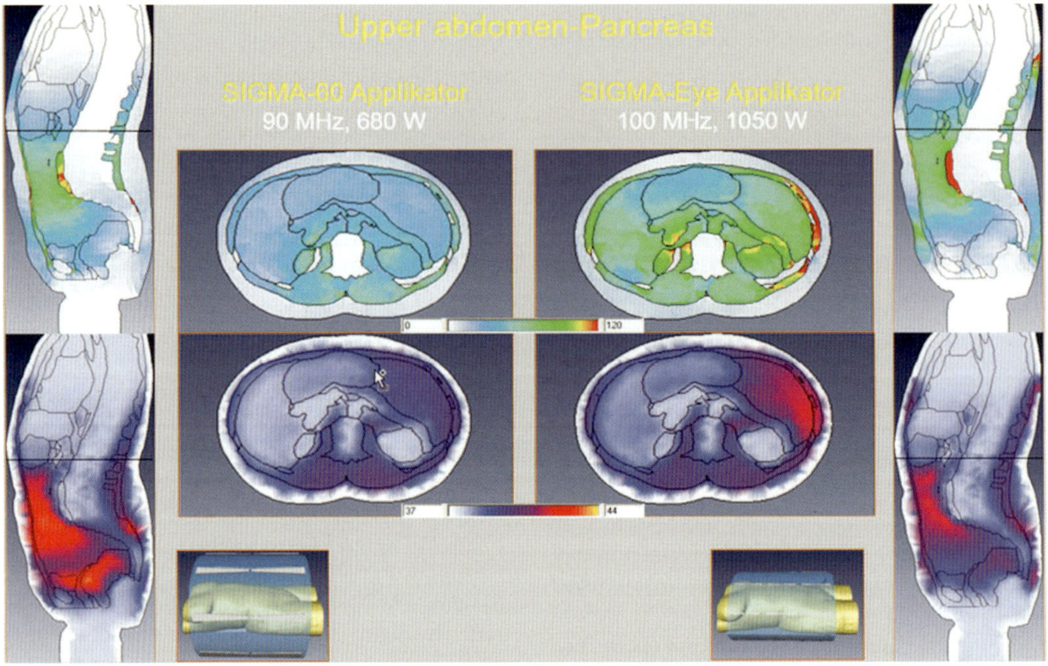

Figure 2.8: SAR distribution (upper row) and temperature distribution (lower row) on a transversal slice of upper abdomen including pancreas in a SIGMA-Eye applicator™ (right column) and SIGMA-60 applicator™ (left column) (Photo provided by Prof. Peter Wust, Charitè-Berlin).

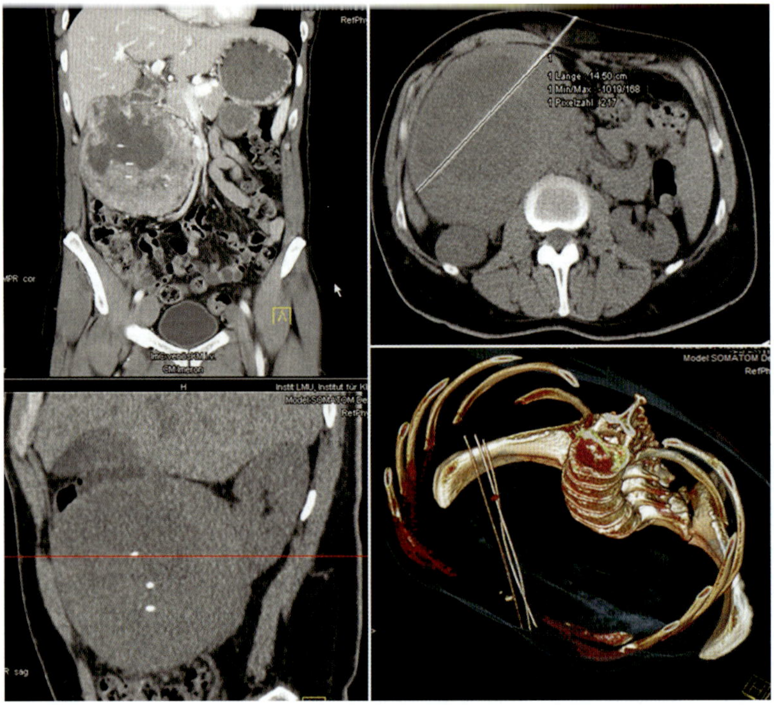

Figure 2.9: Computed tomography (CT) image from a patient with a retroperitoneal leiomyosarcoma, as a representative example of invasive temperature measurements in the upper abdomen.

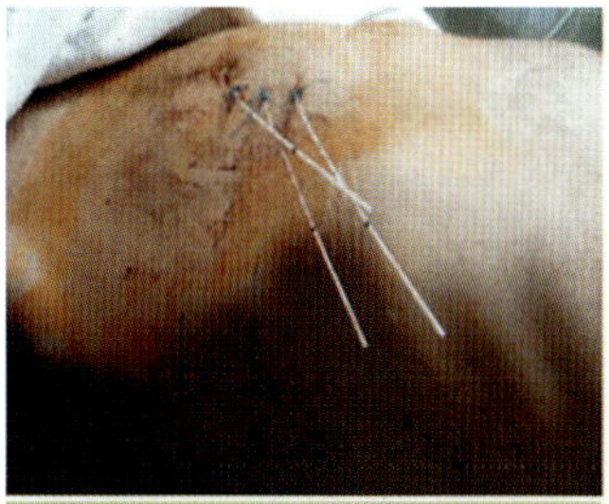

Technical parameter	
Max. power	800 W
Applicator	Sigma-Eye
Frequency	102 MHZ
Target	(-4,-4)

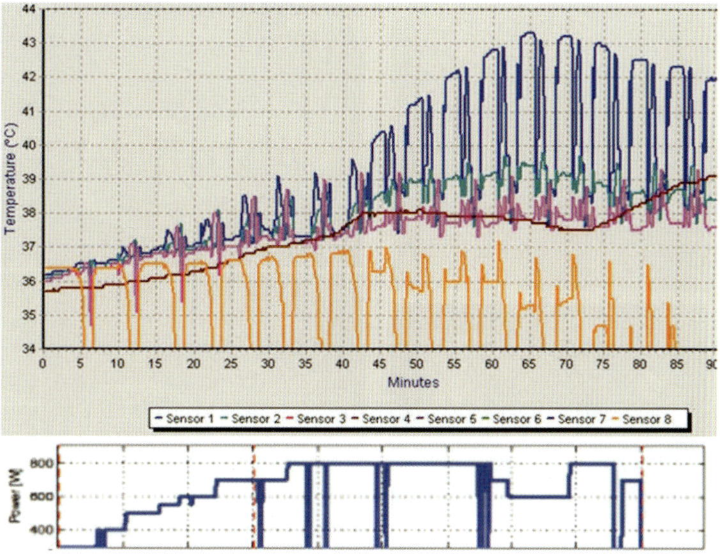

Figure 2.10: Temperature-time-curve (*upper curve*) and power curve (*lower curve*) during a regional deep hyperthermia treatment with invasive temperature measurement (*left image*).

matic representation of the antennas in both applicators.

Figure 2.8 shows the differences between the SIGMA-Eye and the SIGMA-60 applicator on a transversal slice of the upper abdomen, including pancreas, using the treatment planning system *SigmaHyperPlan*™ (Dr. Sennewald Medizintechnik GmbH, Munich, Germany). There is a more homogenous distribution of the specific absorption rate (SAR) and of the achieved higher temperatures in the region of interest using a SIGMA-Eye applicator than using a SIGMA-60 applicator. Moreover, the multi-antenna arrangement in the SIGMA-Eye applicator enables a larger treatment volume; e.g., the whole peritoneum including the liver. The elliptical shape of the SIGMA-Eye applicator provides lower bolus pressure, which makes the treatment more comfortable for the patient. In an intra-patient comparison between both applicators there was no significant difference between temperatures reached in both applicators. Due to the thicker cables in the S-60, the power dissipation is slightly lower than in the S-Eye (approx. 100 W difference). Therefore, the intraluminal temperatures reached at the same amount of applied RF-power in the S-60 are slightly higher than in the S-Eye. On the other hand, the probability of hot spots is lower due to the finer distribution of the E-field through 3-dimensional field control and the longer patient-bolus contact in the S-Eye. If no longitudinal control is necessary, both applicators can be exchanged without loss of quality [7-8].

The treatment of peritoneal carcinomatosis with hyperthermia does not yet provide clinically comparable data with intraperitoneal hyperthermia (HIPEC), but technically this is possible using S-Eye and S-60 applicators. Better SAR distribution than Sigma applicators is provided by the new ALBA system AMC-8. Thermal simulation in a phantom shows a power density of 35-40 W/kg in at least in 50% of peritoneum and a possible thermal enhancement ratio of 1.4-1.5 [9].

To obtain the desired intratumoral temperature with simultaneous protection of the surrounding healthy tissue from heat-induced damage, a three-dimensional temperature measurement of the affected area is required. This can be achieved with the following strategy. If the tumor is located in the pelvic region, intraluminal temperature measurement in the natural orifices such as bladder, rectum or vagina is sufficient because there is a correlation between intraluminal and direct invasive measured temperature in the tumor in the pelvic region [10-11]. If the tumor is located outside the pelvis, catheters inserted invasively into the tumor under CT guidance are needed to provide the necessary information about the on-site temperature distribution during RHT treatment, which intra-

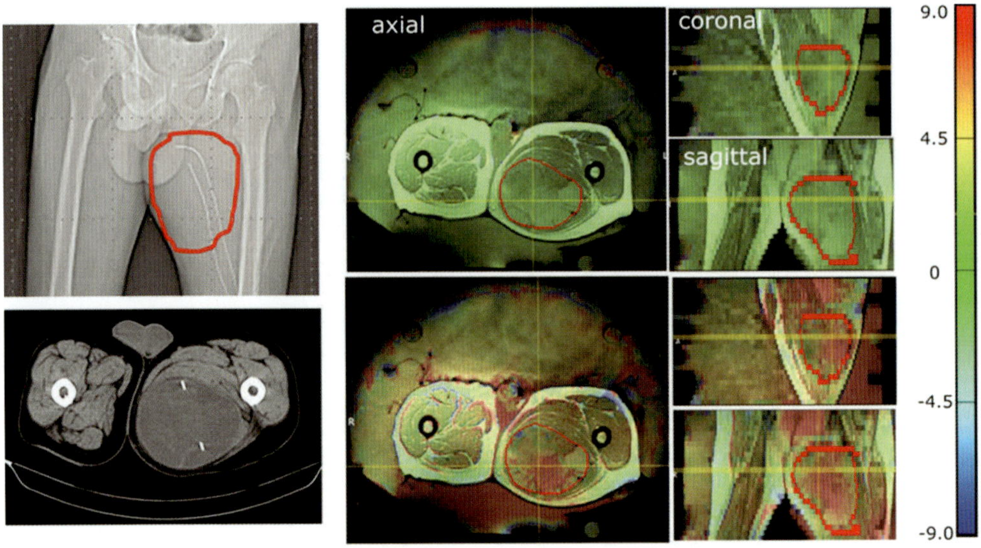

Figure 2.11: Non-invasive and invasive temperature measurement (for validation) with hybrid systems in a soft tissue sarcoma in the left thigh of a male patient.

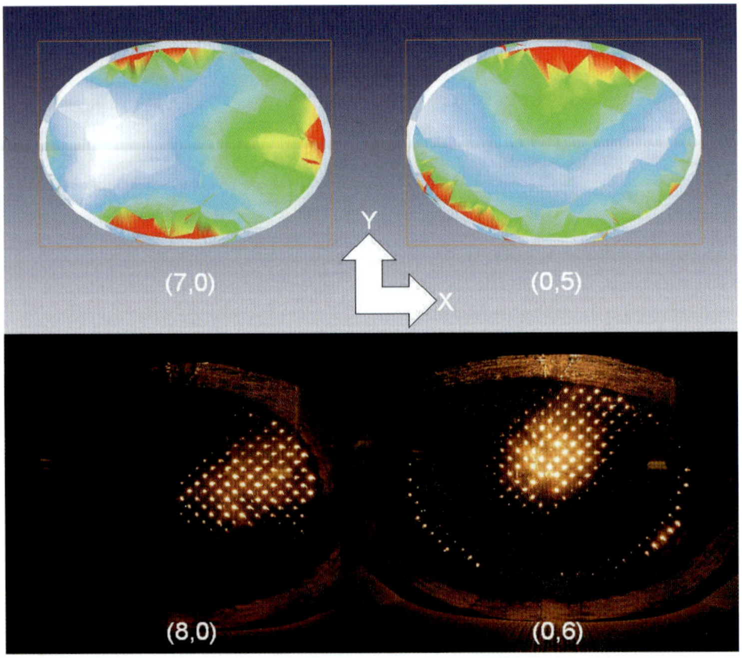

Figure 2.12: According to *SigmaHyperPlan*™ (upper row), the focused RF energy depicted as a green spot moves to the right and upper edge of SIGMA-Eye applicator if the focus is set as (7.0) and (0.5), respectively. In comparison, lamp phantom measurements (lower row) show the results of (8.0) and (0.6). In general, the X value ranges from –8 to 8 and Y from –6 to 6 for RHT treatments using SIGMA-Eye applicator.

luminal temperature measurement cannot provide. However, the implantation of catheters for invasive temperature-measuring requires prior patient consent.

The invasive temperature catheters are clearly visible and a maximum temperature of 43.2°C in the tumor was measured (☞ Figure 2.10). However, as catheters are inconvenient to patients and could cause complications, such as infection or bleeding [12], alternative non-invasive methods for temperature measurement with hybrid systems, consisting of a magnetic resonance (MR) scanner in combination with a Sigma-Eye applicator, have been clinically established (University Hospitals of Berlin, Munich, Erlangen, Tübingen, Rotterdam and Düsseldorf) to provide on-line temperature monitoring during a hyperthermia treatment [8]. Noninvasive temperature measurement in the abdomen is still difficult due to motion artifacts. Hybrid systems enhance the treatment quality by detection of tumor position in the applicator and "hot spots" within healthy tissue [13].

The standard technical parameters depend on the patient's weight and height. They can be defined as follows:

- Forward power: 500-800 W on SIGMA-60 and SIGMA-Eye applicator
- Patient with an anterior-posterior extension of more than 25 cm should be treated with the SIGMA-60, other patients with the SIGMA-Eye or elliptical SIGMA-60 applicator
- Focus range: X coordinate from –8 to 8, Y coordinate from –6 to 6 on SIGMA-Eye applicator (☞ Figure 2.12)
- If possible, none of the applicator's antennas, especially the S-60, should be completely switched off.

The recommended therapy parameters are as follows:

- Mean SAR: 40-70 W/kg
- Maximum intratumoral temperatures: 44°C
- Assumed perfusion: 20 ml/100 g/min
- Reference (vaginal or rectal temperature) temperatures: 42°C
- Position of applicator middle point must be in the center of the longitudinal tumor extension (☞ Figure 2.12)

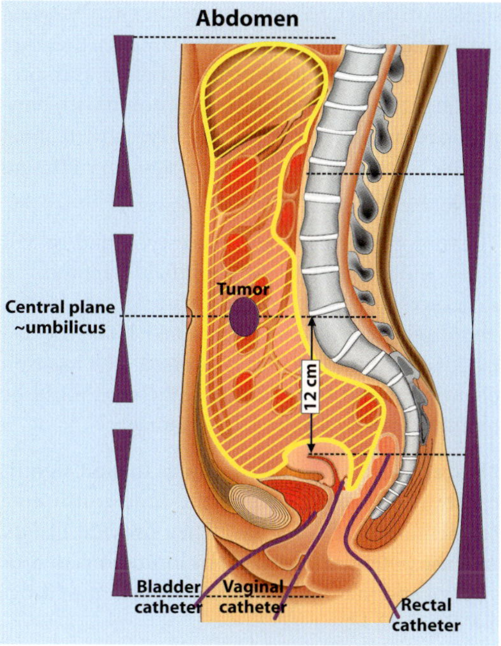

Figure 2.13: Position of applicator (left: SIGMA-Eye; right: SIGMA-60) with respect to an abdominal tumor: The middle point of the applicator is positioned on the navel. (Modified after Prof. Peter Wust, Charitè-Berlin).

The above-mentioned parameters represent the minimum requirements of quality standards.

The positioning of the applicator on the patient should be guided by the CT or MRI scan that clearly indicates the tumor margins and their relation to anatomical points on the patient's surface.

The objectives of these recommendations for hyperthermia procedures as quality assurance guidelines are as follows:

- Treatment planning
- Treatment
- Treatment documentation
- Requirements and characterization of equipment
- Safety aspects
- Hyperthermia staff requirements

2.2.1. Treatment Planning

Before planning a hyperthermia treatment, exclusion and inclusion criteria must be defined and ensured that the patient fulfils the protocol requirements. The patient must be afebrile when starting the treatment and no open wounds (e.g. burn, abscess, skin defect, recent surgery scar) may be present. In the case of healing/healed wounds, these are to be documented with pictures before and after treatment and these must be monitored with temperature measurement probes. The patient must be able to communicate or be responsive after an analgesic sedation [1-3].

The tumor must be localized using CT and/or MR scans and its relation to identifiable anatomical structures of the individual patient, e.g. navel, symphysis etc. has to be determined. Next, the distance to the tumor center is assessed. The location of intratumoral temperature catheters should be indicated clearly on the CT/MR image.

3D-treatment planning continues to gain significance in the clinic, despite the time-consuming segmentation of CT-scans. They provide insight into the potential as well as the limitations of SAR control and may help to define the system settings (☞ Figure 2.12).

For a given hyperthermia system, dimensions of the effective heating fields in perpendicular direction to the patient's longitudinal axis should be estimated from published or measured in-house SAR or temperature distributions in appropriate phantoms. In general, maximum tumor coverage will be obtained if the patient is positioned with respect to the hyperthermia applicator so that as much of the tumor as possible lies between the 50% iso-SAR points along the respective directions. In a hyperthermia applicator it is important that air spaces between applicator wall and patient surface be minimized and - if possible - eliminated. Once the patient is positioned within the applicator, "fine tuning" of patient-applicator position can be done through measurement of electric field intensities on the patient's surface. The E-Field sensors are placed at anterior-central, posterior-central, left-lateral and right-lateral positions on the surface area of interest. Measurements of surface E-fields at low power levels (100-200 W) can guide adjustments of the patient's position within the applicator ring, and reduce the severity of possible hot spots in the skin and subcutaneous tissues during hyperthermia treatment. Such adjustments can also lead to improved tumor heating.

Numerical simulations solve differential equations to calculate the electromagnetic field to achieve power distribution and heat transfer problems for phased array systems. There are several commercial software packages available, such as Sigma Hyperplan (Dr. Sennewald Medizintechnik GmbH, Munich, Germany) or Plan2Heat (UMC Amsterdam, the Netherlands). It should be noted that these packages are still under research development and need to be certified.

The use of hyperthermia treatment planning software helps the operator to achieve the optimum settings for the amplitude and phase parameters. Here fore, a 3D patient model must be created by contouring different tissues derived from CT or MRI images. For a correct simulation, the size of the Image data set in Z-direction should be at least the size of the applicator length (approximately 50-55 cm). The segmentation can be time consuming especially when MRI images are used. Contrast inhomogeneities are a challenge even for Deep

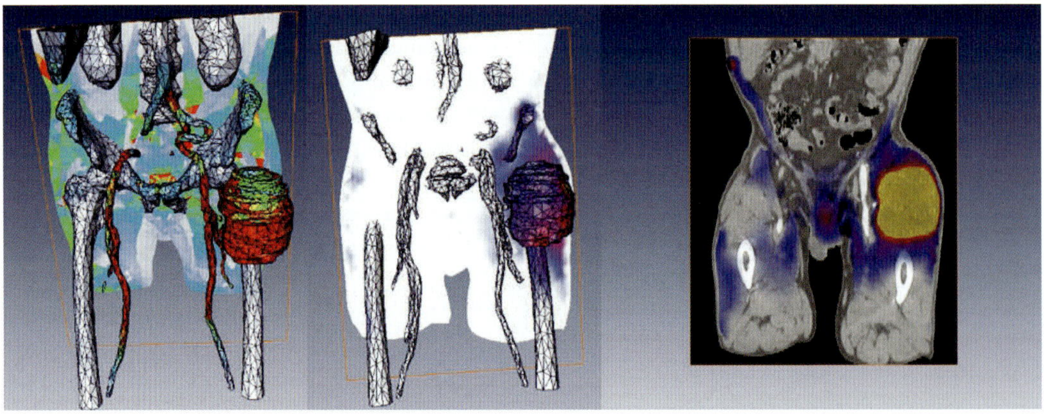

Figure 2.14: Coronal sections of a patient model, location of soft tissue sarcoma in the upper leg region. From left to right: SAR-distribution (red areas display high SAR-rate, temperature distribution (yellow area shows T >42°C).

Learning Algorithms to achieve a good result in an automatic way.

Nevertheless, integrating treatment planning software into the clinical routine should be the gold standard for regional deep and superficial hyperthermia treatments covering all anatomic locations. According to our clinical experience in more than 18.000 treatments in the last 30 years, we have developed an alternative treatment planning work flow which can easily be incorporated into the clinical routine for a large number of patients per day. This guideline has been empirically tested in numerous phantom measurements during the last 30 years and verified by invasive intratumoral temperature measurements in more than 200 patients and has proven to be an effective treatment planning method in clinical operations.

The identification of tumor volume from CT or MRI images ideally requires patient positioning to be identical to the treatment position inside the applicator. The central slice of the tumor volume in the transversal plane is selected (☞ Figure 2.15). A coordinate system (x and y), with the origin in the middle of the patient's contour, is defined. The x and y value from the origin to the center of the tumor volume is measured.

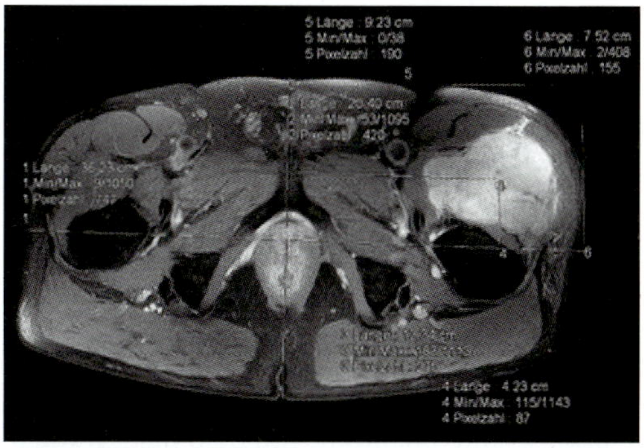

Figure 2.15: Fat-suppressed MRI transversal image showing x(3)/y(4) measurements.

A special formula was developed internally using applicator and phantom data, as well as our clinical experience, to calculate target values.

2.2.2. Treatment Monitoring

Thermometry

- Multisensor probes and/or thermal mapping systems must be used. Preferably one probe is in the tumor or tumor-related site. This probe will be used to define the initial temperature rise and thus the SAR in the tumor area.
- Temperature probes must be positioned endoluminally in bladder, rectum and, if possible, the vagina.
- CT or MR must be used to identify the intratumoral probe positions.
- Power, phase levels and temperatures must be measured at least every minute. In case of mapping systems, a scan must be performed every 5 minutes. If the length of the thermometry track is >15 cm, a scan every 10 minutes is sufficient.

Temperatures and E-field measurements

- All temperatures must be measured by calibrated probes. High resistant metal-free or fiberoptic probes are permitted if calibration determines their inaccuracy to be <0.2°C.
- The tumor temperature goal is 43°C, with higher temperatures (up to maximum 45°C) acceptable depending on the clinical situation. Normal tissue temperatures should not exceed 43-44°C. The thermometry gives no guarantee that higher temperatures will not occur. Prevention of treatment-related pain is the major way to prevent thermal damage to normal tissues.
- Systemic temperature must be monitored at least every 15 minutes orally or via an esophageal probe (in which case the sensor is put on the level of the eighth thoracic vertebrae). Systemic temperature should never exceed 40°C.
- The temperature of the circulating coupling medium (water within the bolus) should also be recorded.
- Initial increase of temperature in the tumor-related sensors should be above 0.2°C/min, but must not exceed 1°C/min.
- Bladder temperature must be controlled and, in case of bladder-toxic chemotherapy regimes, cooled when the temperature rises to >40°C. If the tumor is close to the bladder, it is sufficient to rinse the bladder at 41.5°C to avoid unintentional cooling of the tumor.

- SAR measurement during treatment using in vivo E-field probes and/or thermal pulse techniques is highly recommended and will help to obtain optimal system settings.
- Patient monitoring during RHT treatment: Noninvasive procedures must be used to monitor blood pressure and heart rate every 5 minutes. A more frequent monitoring of the heart rate, for instance through a pulse-oximeter of an ECG monitor which has been made immune from radiofrequency (RF) stray fields, is highly recommended.

Pain

- The patient's anxiety, pain, and general discomfort must be recorded. The location, severity and duration of patient pain, as well as its possible causes and countermeasures taken to alleviate the pain, must be indicated.
- As pain sensation is of major importance for preventing normal tissue damage, analgesic medication should only be used to suppress pre-existing (not power-related) pain from clinically known sites.
- Bolus extension (additional water bags) must be applied if the patient complains about localized pain at the bolus edges.
- Additional cooling to limit the systemic temperature or improve patient comfort should be applied to an extent which is comfortable for the patient, preferably by cooling thorax, forehead and face.

2.2.3. Treatment Documentation

In the protocols, the start and duration of treatment must be defined. A possible definition of the treatment start is the minute in which an intratumoral or tumor-related probe reaches a certain temperature (41.5°C or 42.5°C, depending on the study protocol) or 30 minutes after power has been switched on.

All primary thermometry data must be recorded; however, treatment may be summarized using thermal parameters such as maximum (T_{max}), minimum (T_{min}) and index temperatures (T_{90}, T_{50} and T_{20}) of the tumor. Only if the tumor is close to the rectum, vagina or bladder, the index temperatures of the intraluminal temperatures must be documented.

It is recommended that the following details are recorded on the patient's treatment documentation form:

- Patient and tumor characteristics
- System used, mechanical setup, patient's position, bolus configuration, additional boluses, etc.
- System settings: frequency, phase, amplitude, power (forward and reflected) and any changes during treatment
- Thermometry used and location of temperature probes and mapping tracks
- Possible occurrence of temperature artifacts
- Endoluminal, tumor, normal, systemic and bolus temperatures
- Number of bladder irrigations, if applied
- Hemodynamic parameters, such as heart rate and blood pressure
- Acute toxicities: the occurrence, nature and duration of any discomfort and pain and whether the pain is related to power, bolus pressure or patient positioning
- The occurrence of treatment-limiting factors and discontinuation of treatment, if applicable, and its causes

2.2.4. Requirements and Characterization of Equipment

- The accuracy of the equipment used in the amplitude, phase and power verification procedures must be verified by an independent measurement method.
- A phase accuracy of the heating system of 10°C at the applicator(s) feed point must be obtained.
- An accuracy of the absolute power level of 10% of the actual value must be obtained.
- System performance must be checked regularly using a lamp phantom with bulb matrix, where phase and amplitude settings, phantom positions and bolus configurations are varied [14-15]. During the periodic machine services, additional tests using network analyzers must be performed. This can also help correct skewed focusing.
- The accuracy of patient positioning should be within 1 cm.
- A schedule for periodic system maintenance and control must be present and a logbook must be kept.

- All temperature probes must be calibrated against a temperature standard which is accurate up to ±0.1°C and traceable to a national standard. This calibration could be done weekly by using at least two calibrated mercury thermometers and a stirred water bath with appropriate temperature uniformity and stability.
- The positioning of the thermal mapping technique should be checked periodically. The accuracy of multisensor positions should be checked periodically as well.

2.2.5. Safety Aspects

Safety devices should be incorporated to prevent overheating of the patient. In case of thermometry or computer failure, the heating system should be shut off automatically.

A good audible and visual contact with the patient must be established. The patient provides essential information with regard to power-steering control and his/her general condition. Any information about pain sensation, discomfort or other feelings related to the RHT treatment must be directly forwarded to the treatment team.

Densely clustered surgical clips or metal implants in the treatment area represent reasons to omit RHT treatment [16]. Patients with pacemakers can only be treated if they have an extremity tumor, and, if treated, great caution must be taken. Some centers generally exclude these patients from regional hyperthermia treatments.

The presence of ascites or any other liquid formation in the treatment area is an exclusion criterion for RHT treatment. Larger seromas within the treatment area must be punctured prior to treatment.

2.2.6. Hyperthermia Staff Requirements

For RHT treatments, the responsible staff must consist of a physician, a physicist or physical engineer and a nurse [1-2]. Because of the impact of deep hyperthermia on the physiological condition of the patient; i.e., core temperature, pulse rate, blood pressure and pain, continuous supervision by the physician is highly recommended to ensure patient safety.

2.2.7. References

1. Bruggmoser G, Bauchowitz St, et al. Guideline for the clinical application, documentation and analysis of clinical studies for regional deep hyperthermia, Strahlenther Onkol 2012;[Suppl 2]188:198-211

2. Bruggmoser G, Bauchowitz St, et al. Quality Assurance for Clinical Studies in Regional Deep Hyperthermia, Strahlenther Onkol 2011;187:605-10

3. Lagendijk JJW, Van Rhoon GC, Hornsleth SN, Wust P, De Leeuw ACC, Schneider CJ, Van Ddk JDP, Van Der Zee J, Van Heek-Romanowski R, Rahman SA, Gromoll C. 'Esho Quality Assurance Guidelines for Regional Hyperthermia', International Journal of Hyperthermia, 1998:14:2:125-133.

4. Issels RD, Prenninger SW, Nagele A, et al. Ifosfamide plus etoposide combined with regional hyperthermia in patients with locally advanced sarcomas: a phase II study. J Clin Oncol 1990;8:1818-1829.

5. Thrall DE, LaRue SM, Yu D, et al. Thermal dose is related to duration of local control in canine sarcomas treated with thermoradiotherapy. Clin Cancer Res 2005; 11:5206-5214.

6. Wust P, Hildebrandt B, Sreenivasa G et al. Hyperthermia in combined treatment of cancer. Lancet Oncol 2002;3:487-497.

7. Abdel-Rahman S, Santl M, Futschik G, Köhler B, Wang T, Issels RD. Comparison between the Sigma-Eye and Sigma-60 applicator, Abstract congress of European Society of Hyperthermic Oncology; 2005

8. Fatehi D, Van der Zee J, Van Rhoon G. Intra-patient comparison between two annular array applicators, Sigma-60 and Sigma-Eye: Applied RF power and intraluminally measured temperatures, Int J Hyperthermia 2011;27(3): 214-223.

9. Kok P, Beck M, Löke D et al. Locoregional hyperthermia to enhance the effectiveness of chemotherapy in patients with peritoneal carcinomatosis: a simulation study comparing different locoregional heating systems, Int J Hyperthermia 2020;37(1):76-88.

10. Wust P, Gellermann J, Harder C et al. Rationale for using invasive thermometry for regional hyperthermia of pelvic tumors. Int J Radiat Oncol Biol Phys 1998; 41:1129-1137.

11. Fatehi D, Van der Zee J, Notenboom A, Van Rhoon G. Comparison of intratumor and intraluminal temperatures during locoregional deep hyperthermia of pelvic tumors, Strahlenther Onkol 2007;183(9):479-86.

12. Strobl F, Azam H, Schwarz J B, PaprottkaPh, Geith T, Abdel-Rahman S. et al, CT fluoroscopy-guided closed-tip catheter placement before regional hyperthermia treatment of soft tissue sarcomas: 5-Year experience in

35 consecutive patients, Int J Hyperthermia 2016;32(2): 151-58.

13. Wust P, Gellermann J, Seebass M et al. Teilkörperhyperthermie mit einem Radiofrequenz-multiantennen-Applikator unter on-line Kontrolle in einem 1,5 t MR-Tomographen. Fortschr Röntgenstr 2004;176:363-374.

14. Wust P, Fahling H, Jordan A et al. Development and testing of SAR-visualizing phantoms for quality control in RF hyperthermia. Int J Hyperthermia 1994;10:127-142.

15. Wust P, Fahling H, Felix R, et al. Quality control of the SIGMA applicator using a lamp phantom: a four-centre comparison. Int J Hyperthermia 1995;11:755-767; discussion 867, 869.

16. Lee ER, Sullivan DM, Kapp DS. Potential hazards of radiative electromagnetic hyperthermia in the presence of multiple metallic surgical clips. Int J Hyperthermia 1992;8:809-817.

2.3. Quality Assurance

In order to judge the quality of hyperthermia treatment, it is important to determine the thermal dose delivered during the treatment session. A standardized thermal dose matrix is not available yet. However, the premise of current clinical hyperthermia is that the proven effectiveness of the treatment relies exclusively on its thermal effect on tumors, which is then dependent on temperature and time [1, 2]. Similar to dosimetry in radiotherapy, the objective of Quality Assurance (QA) procedures is to characterize heating devices, confirming adequate heating for the intended applications, as well as to ensure uniform execution of hyperthermia treatments and clinical trials.

2.3.1. Heat Dosimetry

Unlike in isolated tumor cells *in vitro*, solid tumors have connective tissue and vasculature, which can react to the application of heat by changing their function and perfusion, and thus prevent a homogeneous heat dose *in vivo*. Surrounding healthy tissue reacts to heat application, depending on the temperature levels of hyperthermia, with perfusion increase (<42-43°C) or breakdown of perfusion by coagulation (>42-43°C). For this reason, comparable to a radiotherapy dose prescription, the temperature in a certain percentage of the tumor volume is described as the thermal dose, which is specifically expressed by index temperatures T_X. X is the indicated percentage of the tumor volume in which the index temperature exists. For example, T_{50} describes the temperature reached in 50% of the tumor, T_{10} is the temperature reached in at least 10% of the tumor (close to the maximum temperature), and T_{90} is the temperature which is reached in at least 90% of the tumor. It is important to note that this parameter alone does not convey any information about how long the temperature persisted.

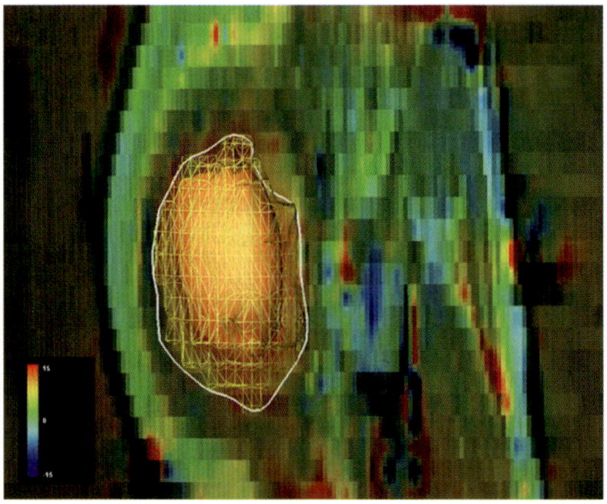

Figure 2.16: Non-invasive MRI-based sagittal thermography of a patient with soft tissue sarcoma in the gluteus maximus muscle. The white line represents the extent of the gross tumor in visualized slice. The yellow grid surface describes T_{90} with a therapeutic temperature elevation of +7.4 degrees (44.4°C). The smaller orange surface displays T_{50} with +11.7 degrees absolute temperature increase (48.7°C).

Due to tumor heterogeneity and increased perfusion (down-cooling) in certain areas, the tumor usually does not experience a homogeneous temperature distribution. Therefore, the T_{90} has been regarded as the most important index temperature that may correlate best with treatment outcome. Nevertheless, the invasive temperature measurement brings such challenges (e.g., accuracy, good spatial coverage, sampling rate), that there is no reason to favor T_{10}, T_{50}, or T_{90}[3]. In addition to the index temperature, the duration of a hyperthermia treatment is also important for effectiveness. For this reason, we can calculate the cumulative minutes, in which a certain T_{90} has been reached during the entire therapy series (including all applied hyperthermia fractions).

The most of thermal dose–effect relationship studies use the equivalent of minutes at 43°C ($CEM_{43°C}$) to predict the cytotoxic effect. It is a convenient method to convert the history of the temperature profile into a single number and can be calculated with the help of the Arrhenius equation:

$$CEM_{43°C} = t \cdot R^{(T-43)}$$

t = time of heat in minutes, T= temperature reached in time t, $R = 2$ for temperatures (T) >43°C, $R = 4$ for temperatures (T) ≤43°C.

If the temperature in the tumor is ≤43°C, the time must be extended per degree by factor 4 to get the same cytotoxic effect. If the temperature is >43°C, the time per degree can be shortened to a half, in order to obtain the same cytotoxic effect. However, other variables, like inflow of oxygen or chemotherapeutics as well as the enhancement of chemotherapeutic effectiveness, are not included in this calculation. Although widely used, this concept holds a number of weaknesses when used as predictor of treatment efficacy. Franckena et al. [4] proposed a thermal dose parameter, TRISE, which they defined as a product of T_{50} rise >37°C normalized to 450 minutes – the total time of all performed treatment sessions. The recent analysis in an independent separate patient cohort shown that both $CEM_{43°C T90}$ and TRISE had a significant effect on local control [2]. The most recent effort to define a uniform, quality controlled and easily quantifiable parameter for reporting and comparison of treatment outcomes with HT plus RT and/or CT during the clinical practice was made by Datta et al. [5], who suggested the temperature–time area under the curve (AUC) during each HT session for T>39°C. The AUC >39°C is a simple, mathematically computable parameter that seems to realistically capture the multifactorial effects of HT across the entire temperature range of 39°C to 45°C and help to fill the void in thermal dose prescription in clinical HT. Its predictive ability remains to be evaluated in prospective studies in a larger patient cohort.

2.3.2. The Hyperthermia QA Guidelines and Their Principles

The current guidelines for superficial, interstitial, and deep hyperthermia [6-9] were produced with the goal to establish a single uniform level of QA and control in HT treatments delivered in all multi-institutional studies. They are related to technical and clinical aspects of QA in hyperthermic oncology and are further supported by well-rounded education guideline papers, including staff requirements, clinical training, wellbeing of the patient [10] and treatment planning [11]. This arsenal of QA guidelines aims to elevate the quality of HT treatments and thus improve patient care. Here we summarize the general concepts and procedures to characterize heating devices for different HT techniques that can further assist the clinical decision and treatment planning processes.

Characterization of the heating performance of HT equipment is based on temperature (rise) measurements and simulations in homogeneous muscle tissue-equivalent phantoms. The methodology was developed to provide easy procedures for QA and to robustly demonstrate the technical performance of deep HT devices in a reproducible manner. For each HT technique, specific criteria and supporting quantities as well as experimental setups have been defined, as summarized in Figure 2.17. For all techniques, the measurements should be carried out at room temperature, i.e. phantom models and water bolus should be at equilibrium with room temperature at the start of each experiment. To prevent manipulation of a heating pattern, the liquid circulating in the water bolus should be kept at room temperature. The thermal assessment during the experiments is done with at least 5 temperature probes situated at prescribed locations and an additional equipment capturing thermal profiles. Temperature distributions in phantoms achieved with superficial and interstitial devices can be easily accessed with an IR camera, while so called LED/lamp phantoms are used for quick, qualitative evaluation of deep devices.

A fundamental criterion to determine whether a heating device is adequate for superficial or interstitial HT is if a temperature rise (TR) of at least 6°C above the starting temperature can be achieved in 6 minutes at 1 cm depth or in 0.5 cm distance, respectively, in a prescribed muscle-tissue equivalent phantom. For deep hyperthermia in head and neck or extremities, the same criterion (TR of 6°C in 6 minutes) is prescribed at the center of the target volume of a homogeneous cylindrical phantom with dimensions appropriate for these body regions, while the systems aiming for deep heating in pelvis, abdomen, and thorax, are considered appropriate when the required temperature increase of 6°C can be achieved in 10 minutes. Apart from the TR criterion, devices intended for deep heating must fulfill an additional requirement on the ability to focalize and steer the heating. In addition to these criteria, supporting performance indicators are essential as they characterize each individual applicator, thus equip the user with information about the capability of the applicator to technically achieve the controlled heating of the specific target volume to the required temperature and thermal dose range. These characteristics, being HT technique specific, help to establish the maximum size and depth of tumors that can be heated adequately by a particular device. The supporting performance indicators are described below for three different types of HT.

Superficial HT

Knowledge about the maximum size and depth of tumors that can be heated adequately is critical for the application of superficial HT. Therefore, two quality indicators related to this information can be derived from temperature rise (TR) measurements in a block phantom (consisting of 9 cm of muscle topped by 1 cm of fat), with prescribed dimensions. The **Thermal Effective Field Size (TEFS)** is defined as the area within the 50% of maximum TR contour (i.e. $\Delta T \geq 3°C$) in the horizontal plane 1 cm under the aperture. Similarly, the **Thermal Effective Penetration Depth (TEPD)** is defined as the depth at which the maximum TR is 50% of the maximum TR (i.e. $\Delta T \geq 3°C$ in 6 minutes) at 1 cm depth.

The horizontal plane at 1 cm depth must always be measured by an IR camera, using a horizontally split phantom with a top layer of 1 cm, which is removed for the IR temperature measurement.

Interstitial HT

The implant/applicator is usually characterized as a single device, but clinically applied in an array of applicators. Therefore, the prescribed procedures aim at verification of both. Analogous to the superficial parameters, the **Effective Heat Length (EHL)** is defined as the length at which the TR is 50% or more of the maximum TR (i.e., temperature difference $\Delta T \geq 3°C$) obtained a constant distance of 5mm from the applicator. Furthermore, it is important to verify to which degree applicators are performing independently, regarding the heating pattern and power output of each applicator.

Deep regional HT (DHT)

The accurate physical characterization includes information about the maximum heating volume of a deeply located target that is achievable with the applicator operating at all frequencies relevant for clinical use. **The Thermal Effective Field Volume (TEFV)** is defined as the volume of a generic phantom enclosed by the 75% maximum temperature rise contour (i.e., $\Delta T \geq 4.5°C$ for a TR of 6°C).Current clinical deep applicators consist of (multiple) rings of antennas arranged symmetrically, and therefore the heating focus is decribed by the **Focus symmetry (FSym)** – the maximum relative (%) deviation of ΔT between the measurements per-

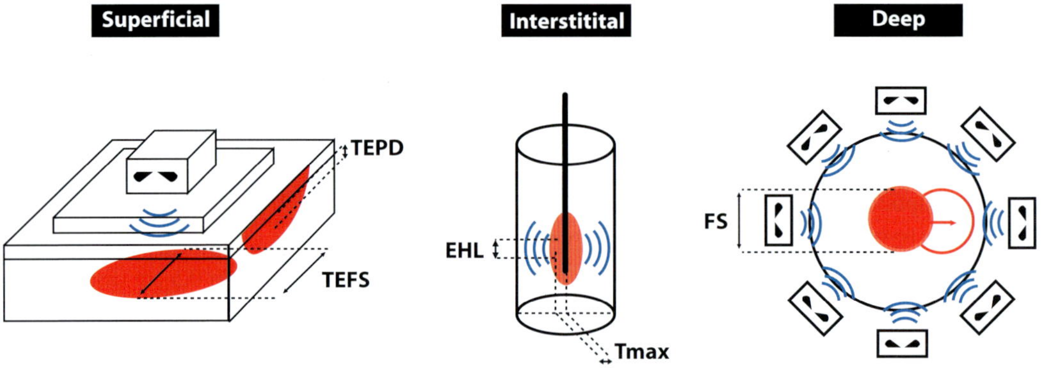

Figure 2.17: QA setups and qualities specified for various HT techniques. This is an open access figure distributed under the CC BY 4.0. Reprinted with permission from HDT; n.d. Available from: http://www.esho.info/.

formed in the four catheters equidistant to the focus isocenter in the radial plane (+/–x and +/–y). The ability to accurately move the heating region isocenter is quantified by the **Focus steering (FSteer)** in terms of precision (mm) between the planned isocenter set in the DHT control software and the experimental maximum temperature location retrieved from the interpolated temperature data. To quickly assess the latter parameters, i.e. the symmetry and steering ability, the use of cylindrical or elliptical LED or Lamp phantoms is recommended, as illustrated in Figure 2.17.

Please note that the QA guidelines for accurate physical characterization of deep heating systems are currently in a submission process and will be subject to minor changes.

2.3.3. Thermometry and Verification

Temperature monitoring is required for effective application of hyperthermia (HT) therapy. It can be used for the optimization of HT settings during treatment as well as for the prediction of treatment efficacy. Furthermore, continuous temperature control gives information about eventual malfunction of the equipment and about tumor changes during therapy (e.g., changes in perfusion, positioning errors, and errors in the treatment planning model) that can be used for a real-time regulation of the treatment. Greater temporal and spatial resolution of the temperature measurement provides better control over the therapy settings and gives more accurate prediction of the treatment outcome.

During HT, temperature should be measured continuously to determine thermal dose described typically by index temperatures and cumulative equivalent minutes at 43°C. For this calculation, it is necessary to measure temperatures inside the tumor. This can be done invasively (directly in the tumor), minimally invasively in predefined body cavities (e.g. the rectum) in contact with or in the proximity to the tumor, or non-invasively. For invasive temperature measurements, catheters are inserted into the tumor by operation or by interventional radiology. For correct determination of T_{90}, catheters must transverse as much of the tumor as possible, ideally through its center, in order to provide a point matrix of temperature. The more measurement points, the more valid are the index temperatures and the equivalent minutes at 43°C computed from this information. However, the risk of side effects, like the risk of bleeding and infections, increases with the number of catheters that are inserted invasively. A convenient minimally invasive technique that can be used for certain tumors and often provided sufficient information about the quality of therapy is the use of endoluminal catheters. However, the correct determination of the T_{90} and $CEM_{43°C}$ is not provided by this procedure. The effect of the therapy with minimally-invasive endoluminally acquired data can be calculated, but the temperatures are usually lower than with invasive measurements.

Temperature can be monitored by means of different physical methods. Thermocouples, fiber-optical sensors or high resistance thermistors are all used for thermometry. The 3D-temperature profiles can then be acquired using multi-sensor probes or thermal mapping, where single-sensor probes are robotically moved every 5-10mm to map the temperature profile along the catheter. The decision regarding a specific thermometry method depends on the simplicity of handling, the price, and (according to the physical compatibility of temperature measurement) the temperature induction method used for HT. For example, when thermocouples are being used, the radio/microwave-frequency hyperthermia must be temporarily switched off during the temperature acquisition. Fiber-optical sensors are susceptible to artifacts in laser heating if the probe is placed near the laser.

The reluctance of the clinicians to place interstitial thermometry catheters remains an important factor of wide clinical acceptance of HT. To provide real-time 3D thermometry feedback, non-invasive thermometry has been subject of research for many years, with MR thermometry being the clinically most advanced temperature measurement method with the highest temporal and spatial resolution. Due to relative nature of this technology, where the temperature change is relative to a baseline condition, the accuracy of MR thermometry is affected by blood flow and motion (i.e., breathing, bowel and cardiac motion). Therefore, MR thermometry is clinically applied for tumor locations where measurements are not strongly affected by such artifacts, e.g., soft tissue sarcomas and tumors in extremities. Under such circumstances, MR thermometry yields an accuracy of ~1°C.

2.3.5. Future Aspects

The majority of clinical trials have shown a significant clinical benefit of adding hyperthermia (HT) to chemo- and/or radiotherapy. As a result, the application of almost all HT techniques has been growing steadily during the past two decades. Apart from historically more traditional use of RF/MW devices, a steep rise in application of perfusion-based technologies HIPEC and HIVEC is evident [12]. To achieve HT treatment goals, accurate treatment planning and delivery are crucial and have been major topics of research for the past two decades. Hyperthermia treatment planning (HTP) serves, e.g., to design new applicators, to test novel treatment approaches in silico, and to provide insight in treatment safety. HTP is the process in which the multidisciplinary HT team defines the optimal treatment plan for a specific cancer patient, using the available HT treatment resources. The HTP has matured and is being regularly used for pre-treatment planning as well as for real-time guidance. Apart from researching even better and faster treatment optimization algorithms, the most admirable advance of high clinical importance is the methodology of calculating the beneficial effect of HT in radiotherapy dose enhancement. In this radiobiological modeling, radiosensitization effect of HT is determined by using an extended version of the LQ-model with temperature-dependent radiosensitivity parameters.

Translating an accurate thermal dose from treatment planning into a clinical therapy session remains extremely challenging, mainly due to unknown thermal and dielectric parameters specific to each patient, but also due to eventual mismatches in patient positioning, bolus shape, or EM signal delivery. Due to the limited knowledge of tissue properties and their physiological dynamics (blood perfusion in particular), HTP still carries uncertainties that may lead to sub-optimal delivery of the HT treatment. Online thermometry feedback is thus essential to monitor treatment quality. Invasive thermometry through temperature probes is currently the gold standard and prescribed by QA guidelines. As these probes provide information only from very few locations and can cause infections [13], noninvasive three-dimensional technology, MR thermometry in particular, is emerging to improve guidance of HT treatments. Besides simultaneous temperature monitoring, MR provides the possibility to determine different physiological measurements, including changes in the treated tissue, like perfusion or the inflow of special medicines in combination with contrast media. Despite its recent development [14], with its current accuracy and susceptibility to motion artifacts, the MR treatment guidance cannot yet substitute temperature probe measurements and serves just as a valuable treatment assistance and retrospective thermal dose estimator. The most advanced high-precision MR-adaptive HT will likely remain a technology used mainly in academic centers for the upcoming decade.

Advances in computational modeling have aided the development of new applicators consisting of high number of antennas operating at higher frequencies, thus providing greater control over the treatment parameters. These devices can induce a smaller heat focus, which can be dynamically adjusted to conformal heating of irregular target regions. Improved spatial control of the energy deposition allows for treatment of (challenging) tumor sites while sparing adjacent critical structures. While the applicators for treatment of deep seated tumors in head and neck have been shown clinically feasible [15], noninvasive heat delivery to treat intracranial tumors [16] has to be further developed before it enters clinical trials.

2.3.6. References

1. Bakker A et al. Temperature and thermal dose during radiotherapy and hyperthermia for recurrent breast cancer are related to clinical outcome and thermal toxicity: a systematic review. Int J Hyperthermia 2019;36(1):1024-1039.

2. Kroesen M et al. Confirmation of thermal dose as a predictor of local control in cervical carcinoma patients treated with state-of-the-art radiation therapy and hyperthermia. Radiother Oncol 2019;140:150-158.

3. van Rhoon GC. Is CEM43 still a relevant thermal dose parameter for hyperthermia treatment monitoring? Int J Hyperthermia 2016;32(1):50-62.

4. Franckena M et al. Hyperthermia dose-effect relationship in 420 patients with cervical cancer treated with combined radiotherapy and hyperthermia. Eur J Cancer 2009;45(11):1969-78.

5. Datta NR et al. Quantification of thermal dose in moderate clinical hyperthermia with radiotherapy: a relook

using temperature-time area under the curve (AUC). Int J Hyperthermia 2021;38(1):296-307.

6. Bruggmoser G et al. Quality assurance for Clinical Studies in Regional Deep Hyperthermia. Strahlenther Onkol 2011;187(10):605-610.

7. Dobšíçek Trefná H et al. Quality assurance guidelines for superficial hyperthermia clinical trials: I. Clinical requirements. Int J Hyperthermia 2017;33(4):471-82.

8. Dobšíçek Trefná H et al. Quality assurance guidelines for superficial hyperthermia clinical trials : II. Technical requirements for heating devices. Strahlenther Onkol 2017;193(5):351-66.

9. Dobšíçek Trefná H et al. Quality assurance guidelines for interstitial hyperthermia. Int J Hyperthermia 2019; 36(1):277-294.

10. Myerson RJ et al. Components of a hyperthermia clinic: recommendations for staffing, equipment, and treatment monitoring. Int J Hyperthermia 2014;30(1): 1-5.

11. Paulides MM et al. ESHO benchmarks for computational modeling and optimization in hyperthermia therapy. Int J Hyperthermia 2021;38(1):1425-1442.

12. Kok HP et al. Heating technology for malignant tumors: a review. Int J Hyperthermia 2020;37(1):711 741.

13. van der Zee J et al. Practical limitations of interstitial thermometry during deep hyperthermia. Int J Radiat Oncol Biol Phys 1998;40(5):1205-12.

14. VilasBoas-Ribeiro I et al. POD-Kalman filtering for improving noninvasive 3D temperature monitoring in MR-guided hyperthermia. Med Phys 2022;49(8):4955-4970.

15. Verduijn GM et al. Deep hyperthermia with the HYPERcollar system combined with irradiation for advanced head and neck carcinoma - a feasibility study. Int J Hyperthermia 2018;34(7):994-1001.

16. Ghaderi Aram M et al. Radiobiological evaluation of combined gamma knife radiosurgery and hyperthermia for pediatric neuro-oncology. Cancers (Basel) 2021; 13(13):3277.

3. Clinical Results of Quality-Assured Hyperthermia

3.1. Hyperthermia Alone

In the perception of many cancer patients, hyperthermia is a treatment comparable to surgery, radio- and chemotherapy. Suffering from a malignant disease and confronted with standard therapy of the established evidence-based oncology, some patients are desperately searching for treatment alternatives. Regional hyperthermia in the temperature range of 40-44°C or fever-like treatment at 39-40 °C seem to be a quite attractive choice to avoid radical surgery, chemo- and/or radiotherapy. Up to date, there are no convincing data for hyperthermia alone in the treatment of any malignancy, including whole body, local, and regional hyperthermia techniques.

This fact remains true despite many contradictory advertisements in the internet. Evidence-based hyperthermia must be used in combination with standard treatments in order to further sensitize the tumor tissue for better oncological outcomes. Therefore, local and regional hyperthermia techniques are *not alternatives* but *additive options* in the treatment of specific cancer diseases as discussed in this book. The role of whole body hyperthermia remains unclear and it should be performed within clinical trials.

3.2. Chemotherapy and Hyperthermia

Several phase II and phase III studies have been completed addressing the role of hyperthermia combined with chemotherapy [1]. More than half of the clinical trials identified in the ClinicalTrials.gov registry focused on the use of hyperthermic intraperitoneal chemotherapy (HIPEC) after radical cytoreductive surgery. Regional hyperthermia using a non-invasive external heating device was the second most used technique followed by whole body hyperthermia and superficial hyperthermia [2].

In this chapter, we describe the more recent developments and the results of selected trials. We also address the specific types of heating technology combining hyperthermia with chemotherapy in the treatment of certain types of malignancies.

3.2.1. Peritoneal carcinomatosis of epithelial ovarian cancer (EOC)

Within more than 15 years, **HIPEC** has been investigated mostly in advanced patients with **peritoneal carcinomatosis** of several malignancies including gastric cancer, malignant mesothelioma, ovarian carcinoma, and pseudomyxoma [3-6]. It is to note that none of these phase II studies, as well as the one completed phase III study in patients with peritoneal carcinomatosis of colorectal cancer [7] were designed to separately evaluate the relative contributions of the cytoreductive surgery and the effect of HIPEC to the improvements in outcome that was observed in some of these early trials. More recently, the additional benefit of HIPEC has been addressed in patients with advanced epithelial ovarian cancer (EOC) in the interval or recurrent setting. The first randomized trial, published by Spiliotis et al. in 2015, showed a 13-month improvement in survival with the addition of HIPEC to secondary cytoreductive surgery, a benefit found in both platinum-sensitive and platinum-resistant cohorts [8]. The phase III study of van Driel et al. randomized women with stage III EOC undergoing neoadjuvant chemotherapy to interval cytoreductive surgery (CRS) with and without HIPEC with cisplatin at a dose of 100 mg/m² [9]. The women who underwent CRS with HIPEC demonstrated a 3.5-month improvement in progression-free survival and a 12-month improvement in overall survival. These findings support the use of HIPEC in this setting, although the trial had significant limitations, including the lack of stratification criteria according to the International Federation of Gynecology and Obstetrics, BRCA mutation status, imbalance between the two groups, and randomization prior to surgery. Despite these limitations, several centers routinely discuss HIPEC with cisplatin at a dose of 100 mg/m² in the interval setting in the subset of patients with abdominally confined disease, whom they anticipate will experience optimal CRS (the removal of all tumors to microscopic disease). An umbrella review including six meta-analyses of HIPEC was recently published. In primary EOC, the combination of HIPEC with interval cytoreductive surgery significantly improved OS (HR=

0.66) and DFS (HR=0.54) compared with CRS alone [10].

In summary, following the ongoing debate and controversial discussion none of the studies in EOC can be unequivocally recommend HIPEC as a new standard treatment of care, despite offering a valid treatment option in selected cases.

3.2.2. Non-muscle-invasive bladder cancer (NMIBC)

Hyperthermic intravesical chemotherapy (HIVEC) has been extensively investigated in patients with non-muscle-invasive bladder cancer (NMIBC), the most prevalent type of bladder cancer. Intermediate and high-risk non- muscle invasive bladder cancer has a 50% risk of recurrence and 20% risk of progression to muscle invasive bladder carcinoma within 5 years, despite the use of intravesical adjuvant treatments (such as BCG or mitomycin C) that are recommended by clinical guidelines [11]. Therefore, optimizing therapeutic strategies are needed. To compare recurrence-free survival (RFS) with adjuvant intravesical mitomycin C (MMC) at normothermia or hyperthermia using the COMBAT bladder recirculation system (Combat Medical, St. Albans, UK) at 43°C for 30 and 60 min, a prospective phase III randomized controlled trial (HIVEC-1) accrued across 13 centers between 2014 and 2020 in Spain [12]. After completing transurethral resection of the bladder and immediate postoperative MMC instillation, patients with IR-NMIBC were randomised (1:1:1) to four weekly followed by three monthly 40 mg MMC instillations at normothermia (control; n= 106), 43°C for 30 min (n=107), or 43°C for 60 min (n=106). Therapeutic compliance was defined as four or more instillations. The primary outcome was RFS at 24 months in the intention-to-treat (ITT) and per-protocol (PP) populations. The secondary outcomes included progression-free survival at 24 months, safety outcome measures, and changes in health-related quality of life. The ITT 24-mo RFS was 77% for control, 82% for 43°C-30 min, and 80% for 43°C-60 min (P=0.6). The PP 24-month RFS was 77% for control, 83% for 43°C-30 min, and 80% for 43°C-60 min (P=0.59). Six patients progressed to muscle-invasive disease in the ITT population (four in the control, one in the 43°C-30 min, and 43°C-60 min groups each) and four in the PP population (all controls). Serious adverse events occurred in 26 patients (8.1%), and we were unable to demonstrate a difference between groups (P=0.5). Adverse events, mainly dysuria and spasms, occurred in 124 patients (33% in control, 35% in 43°C-30 min, and 48% in 43 °C-60 min; P=0.05). The total International Prostate Symptom Score worsened by 1.2 ± 7.3 points, similarly across groups (P=0.29). The Functional Assessment of Cancer Therapy-Bladder domains and indexes showed no significant change. In conclusion, four-month adjuvant hyperthermic MMC using the COMBAT recirculation system for 30 and 60 min in IR-NMIBC was well tolerated, but did not result to be superior to normothermic MMC at 24 months.

HIVEC-II was an open-label, phase II randomized controlled trial of intravesical hyperthermic chemotherapy versus chemotherapy alone in patients with intermediate-risk NMIBC recruited at 15 centers between May 2014 and December 2017 [13]. Patients were randomly assigned (1:1) to adjuvant with mitomycin C at 43°C or to room-temperature mitomycin C. Both treatment arms received six weekly instillations of 40 mg of mitomycin C lasting for 60 min. The primary endpoint was 24-month disease-free survival as determined via cystoscopy and urinary cytology. Analysis was by intention to treat. A total of 259 patients (131 CHT vs 128 control) were randomized. At 24 months, 42 patients (32%) in the CHT group and 49 (38%) in the control group had experienced recurrence. Disease-free survival at 24 months was 61% (95% confidence interval [CI] 51-69%) in the CHT arm and 60% (95% CI, 50-68%) in the control arm (HR=0.92, 95% CI, 0.62-1.37; log-rank P=0.8). Progression-free survival was higher in the control arm (HR=3.44, 95% CI, 1.09-10.82; log-rank P=0.02) on intention-to-treat analysis but was not significantly higher on per-protocol analysis (HR 2.87, 95% CI, 0.83-9.98; log-rank P=0.06). Overall survival was similar (HR 2.55, 95% CI, 0.77-8.40: log-rank P=0.09). Patients undergoing CHT were less likely to complete their treatment (n=75, 59% vs n=111, 89%). Adverse events were reported by 164 patients (87 CHT vs 77 control). Major (grade III) adverse events were rare (13 CHT vs 7 control).

From these results, HIVEC cannot be recommended over chemotherapy alone for intermediate-risk NMIBC. Adverse events following CHT were of low grade and short-lived, although patients were less likely to complete their treatment. HIVEC-I and II were the first published randomized trial to use conductive hyperthermia for NMIBC.

In contrast to conductive hyperthermia, the technology **of radiofrequency-induced thermotherapy effect (RITE)** using the Synergo-System at a radiofrequency (915 MHz) to heat the bladder wall lining **combined with intravesical chemotherapy** (MMC; mitomycin C) seemed to be effective. In a first report by Colombo et al., improvement of recurrence-free survival was seen in a multicenter clinical trial comparing intravesical chemotherapy with mitomycin C alone and combined with local microwave hyperthermia for prevention of recurrence of superficial transitional cell cancer of the bladder [14]. In a randomized trial of 83 patients with intermediate and high-risk NMIBC, RITE resulted in a significantly higher recurrence-free survival (60% vs 20%; P<0.001) in comparison to MMC at median follow-up of 91 months [15]. Another randomized trial of 190 BCG-naïve patients with intermediate or high-risk NMIBC reported that patients with papillary-only disease treated with RITE had significantly better recurrence-free survival compared to those treated with BCG (81.8% vs 64.8%; P=0.02) following per-protocol analysis [16]. However, in the BCG failure setting, the HYMN trial closed early at interim analysis as RITE-treated patients had a lower DFS rate in comparison to the control group [17].

Regional Hyperthermia (**RHT**) and Partial-Body Hyperthermia (**PBH**) are based **upon three-dimensional multi-antenna, microwave applicators** (BSD SIGMA-Eye™ applicator). The applicator can be integrated in a magnetic resonance tomography [18-20]. Non-invasive treatment monitoring is provided by such hybrid systems to characterize temperature as well as perfusion during hyperthermia [21]. The heating pattern can cover larger anatomical regions e.g. full peritoneum (for peritoneal carcinomatosis) or upper abdomen (for liver metastases). There is experience using an **external heating device** with **70 MHz regional hyperthermia (RHT)** and mitomycin C in bladder cancer [22, 23]. The safety and feasibility of this treatment combination **for intermediate and high risk NMIBC** has been published [24]. Between 2009 and 2011, 20 patients were treated with intravesical mitomycin C (40 mg) combined with regional hyperthermia. Treatment consisted of 6 weekly sessions followed by a maintenance period of 1 year with 1 hyperthermia-mitomycin C session every 3 months. Regional hyperthermia was administered using a 70 MHz phased array system with 4 antennas. Toxicity was scored using CTC (Common Toxicity Criteria) 3.0. The records of 18 of 20 patients could be analyzed. Median follow-up was 46 months. Of the 18 patients, 15 (83%) completed the induction period of 6 treatments. Four patients (22%) discontinued treatment because of physical complaints without exceeding grade 2 toxicity. Toxicity scored according to CTC 3.0 was limited to grade 1 in 43% of cases and grade 2 in 14%. Mean T90 and T50 bladder temperatures were 40.6°C and 41.6°C, respectively. The 24-month recurrence-free survival rate was 78%.

In summary, intravesical devices (HIVEC, RITE) or external heating systems (RHT/PBH) in combination with chemotherapy have shown promising efficacy. Considerable heterogeneity in patient cohorts, treatment sessions, use of maintenance regimens, and single-arm study design makes it difficult to draw solid conclusions and results of randomized controlled trials are eagerly awaited.

3.2.3. High-risk soft tissue sarcomas (HR-STS) of adults

The most evidence to prove the role of **regional hyperthermia** has shown in the **combination with neoadjuvant chemotherapy** (NAC) in high-risk soft tissue sarcomas (HR-STS) of adults. Using the current deep regional hyperthermia (RHT) methodology, the European Organization for Research and Treatment of Cancer (EORTC) and the European Society for Hyperthermic Oncology (ESHO) completed a multicentric, large Intergroup phase III trial (EORTC 62961/ESHO RHT-95) in order to define the impact of RHT within a treatment strategy for patients with **primary or recurrent high-risk soft tissue sarcoma** (STS) (>5 cm, grade 2 or 3, deep to the fascia) or for the same group of patients after inadequate surgery [25]. In this trial all patients with high-risk STS, stratified to extremity (E) and to non-extremity (non-E), received systemic NAC chemotherapy (four cycles doxorubicin, ifosfamide, and etoposide) and were randomized in two arms (NAC alone vs. NAC + RHT) followed by definitive surgery and radiotherapy.

Thereafter, an additional four cycles of the NAC regimen were administered with or without RHT, according to the initial randomization. 341 patients were enrolled, with 169 randomly assigned to NAC plus regional hyperthermia and 172 to NAC alone. All patients were included in the analysis of the primary endpoint, and 332 patients who received at least one cycle of chemotherapy were included in the safety analysis. **After a median follow-up of 34 months** (IQR 20-67), 132 patients had local progression (56 NAC plus regional hyperthermia vs 76 NAC). Patients were more likely to experience local progression or death in the NAC-alone group compared with the NAC plus regional hyperthermia group (relative hazard [RH] 0.58, 95% CI, 0.41-0.83; P=0.003), with an absolute difference in LPFS at 2 years of 15% (95% CI 6-26; 76% NAC plus regional hyperthermia vs 61% NAC). For disease-free survival the relative hazard was 0·70 (95% CI, 0.54-0.92, P=0.011) for NAC plus regional hyperthermia compared with NAC alone. The treatment response rate in the group that received regional hyperthermia was 28.8%, compared with 12.7% in the group who received chemotherapy alone (P=0.002). In a prespecified per-protocol analysis of patients who completed NAC plus regional hyperthermia induction therapy compared with those who completed NAC alone, overall survival was better in the combined therapy group (HR 0.66, 95% CI, 0.45-0.98, P=0.038). Leucopenia (grade 3 or 4) was more frequent in the combine group compared with the NAC-alone group (128 of 165 vs 106 of 167, P=0.005). Hyperthermia-related adverse events were pain, bolus pressure, and skin burn, which were mild to moderate in 66 (40.5%), 43 (26.4%), and 29 patients (17.8%), and severe in seven (4.3%), eight (4.9%), and one patient (0.6%), respectively. Two deaths were attributable to treatment in the combined treatment group, and one death was attributable to treatment in the NAC-alone group [25]. To analyze whether the reported local progression-free survival by adding regional hyperthermia to neoadjuvant chemotherapy translates into improved survival, we performed a **long-term analysis after a median follow-up of 11.3 years** [26]. For survival (dead of disease), 329 patients (147 women, 182 men) were eligible for the intention-to-treat analysis. By December 2014, 220 patients (67%; 95% CI, 62-72) had experienced disease relapse, and 188 (57%; 95% CI, 52-62) had died. Compared with NAC alone, adding regional hyperthermia improved local progression-free survival [HR], 0.65; 95% CI, 0.49-0.86; P=0.002). Patients randomized to NAC + RHT chemotherapy had prolonged survival rates compared with those randomized to NAC alone (HR, 0.73; 95% CI, 0.54-0.98; P=0.04) with 5-year survival of 62.7% (95% CI, 55.2-70.1) vs 51.3% (95% CI, 43.7-59.0), respectively, and 10-year survival of 52.6% (95% CI, 44.7-60.6) vs 42.7% (95% CI, 35.0-50.4). **In summary, adding regional hyperthermia to neoadjuvant chemotherapy is a new effective treatment strategy for patients with high-risk STS, including STS with an abdominal or retroperitoneal location** [27].

3.2.4. Localized relapse or metastatic disease of soft-tissue sarcoma

Patients with **local recurrence of soft-tissue sarcoma after anthracycline-based chemotherapy** have a dismal prognosis, particularly when surgery is not possible. To facilitate resection and improve long-term tumor control, an intensified perioperative treatment consisting of ICE (ifosfamide 6 g/m, carboplatin 400 mg/m, and etoposide 600 mg/m) in combination with regional hyperthermia (RHT) was applied to maximize local control. In a previous analysis, including patients with **progressive disease after first-line chemotherapy** combinations, patients who received **systemic ICE chemotherapy (ifosfamide, carboplatin, etoposide) with RHT** showed an objective response rate of 20% [28]. A more extended report on 49 patients confirmed these results. The range of observed response rate was between 17% and 45%, respectively, and was dependent upon the initial pre-treatment failure of chemotherapy either with or without RHT [29].

The results were in the same range as previously reported by the SHOWG phase II trial in a series of patients with **metastatic STS** using a closed radiant heat device (Aquatherm) for **whole-body hyperthermia (WBH)** to raise the patients' core temperature to 41.8°C for 60 minutes. In pretreated patients, the response rate to ICE chemotherapy simultaneously with WBH was 24% [30]. Several phase II studies have been completed with some promising results [31], but the efficacy of radiative WBH combined with chemotherapy has not yet been proven in the scope of a randomized trial. At the borderline of WBH, there is interest to define fever range (39-40°C) whole body hyperthermia (FR-WBH) combined with systemic chemotherapy. New technologies include infra-red radiative antennas (e.g. HT3000 system; Heckel Medizintechnik; Germany). This approach is based on preclinical results in animal models showing stimulation of the immune system [32-34] and an equal anti-tumor efficacy for long durations (4-6 hours, 39-40°C) of FR-WBH, as compared to conventional WBH (1 hour, >41,5°C) [35]. More recently, clinical data of FR-WBH in combination with Il-2, checkpoint inhibition and low-dose chemotherapy in patients with advanced disease including STS have been published [36].

A large monocentric analysis evaluated the efficacy of the second-line strategy in **213 sarcoma patients who had received ICE plus RHT between 1996 and 2018** [37]. Patients aged ≥18 years with locally advanced high-risk STS, either with or without metastasis, treated with ICE + RHT after the failure of first-line anthracycline-based chemotherapy were included. Radiographic response, toxicity, progression-free survival (PFS), and overall survival (OS) were assessed. Of these, 110 patients met the selection criteria (progressive disease, suitable high-grade STS histology, anthracycline pretreatment, RHT treatment) for the analysis. Fifty-four patients had locally advanced disease without metastases (LA-STS), and 56 patients had additional metastatic disease (M-STS). Disease control was achieved in 59% of LA-STS patients and in 47% of M-STS patients. For LA-STS, 21% of the patients achieved radiographic response, facilitating resection in 4 patients (7%), compared with 11% of the M-STS patients, facilitating resection in 5 patients (9%). PFS was significantly longer in LA-STS than in M-STS (10 vs. 4 months, P<0.0001). Median OS was 26 months in LA-STS and 12 months in M-STS. Disease control was the only independent prognostic factor for improved OS in multivariate analysis. Toxicity was high with neutropenic fever occurring in 25% of the patients and three therapy-related deaths (3%). **ICE + RHT demonstrated activity in high-risk STS and facilitated resection in selected patients after anthracycline failure. Disease control was associated with improved OS.**

Isolated limb perfusion for extremity sarcomas or melanomas

Prophylactic hyperthermic isolated limb perfusion (ILP) with **melphalan alone** for the treatment of malignant melanoma was studied in a well-designed large multicenter randomized trial and showed to be of no significant value [38]. However, the situation changes completely by the utilization of **TNF (tumor necrosis factor)** in the ILP setting. TNF plus melphalan-based hyperthermic ILP has been proven to be highly effective in multicenter non-randomized trial settings, demonstrating response rates above 70% and limb salvage rates above 80%, especially in **locally advanced soft tissue sarcomas of the extremities.** This resulted in the approval of TNF in Europe for the ILP setting [39]. Still, no firm conclusion can be drawn for ILP regarding the relative effect of hyperthermia in the combined action with TNF or melphalan. Also, there was no beneficial effect on overall survival reported in these trials.

3.2.5. Pancreatic Cancer

Regional hyperthermia (RHT) with cisplatin added to gemcitabine showed efficacy in gemcitabine-pretreated patients with advanced **pancreatic ductal adenocarcinoma** [40]. Recently, **HEAT** (Hyperthermia European Adjuvant Trial), **a randomized clinical trial** to investigate RHT with cisplatin added to gemcitabine (GPH) compared with gemcitabine (G) in the adjuvant setting of resected pancreatic ductal adenocarcinoma (PDAC) has been completed [41]. The multicenter, open-label trial randomly assigned patients to either GPH (gemcitabine 1000 mg/m² on day 1, 15 and cisplatin 25 mg/m² with RHT on day 2, 3 and 15, 16) or to G (gemcitabine 1000 mg/m² on day 1, 8, 15), four-weekly over six cycles. Disease-free survival (DFS) was the primary endpoint. Secondary endpoints included overall survival (OS) and safety. A total of 117 eligible patients (median age 63 years) were randomly allocated to treatment (57 GPH; 60 G). With a follow-up time of 56.6 months, the median DFS was 12.7 compared to 11.2 months for GPH and G, respectively (P=0.394). Median post-recurrence survival was significantly prolonged in the GPH group (15.3 vs 9.8 months; P=0.031). Median OS reached 33.2 vs 25.2 months (P=0.099) with 5-year survival rates of 28.4% vs 18.7%. Excluding eight patients who received additional capecitabine in the G arm (investigators choice), median OS favored GPH (P=0.052). Adverse events CTCAE grade ≥0.3 occurred in 61.5% (GPH) vs 63.6% (G) of patients. Two patients in the G group died because of treatment-related toxic effects. Although **the randomized study failed to demonstrate a significant difference in DFS, it showed a difference in post-recurrence survival and a trend for improved OS** [41]. The results should be discussed in patients with recurrent local and distant disease after standard chemotherapy (e.g., m-FOLFIRINOX, gemcitabine plus nab-paclitaxel) whether RHT with cisplatin added to gemcitabine (GPH) offers a treatment option for these patients.

3.2.6. Breast Cancer

Patients with **triple-negative primary breast cancer (TNBC),** who have residual invasive carcinoma after neoadjuvant chemotherapy, have poor prognosis. Proven adjuvant approaches to reduce the risk of recurrence and improve outcome in patients with non-pathological complete response (non-pCR) are limited. From an institutional registry, a consecutive case series of patients with operable, unilateral, primary invasive non-inflammatory early TNBC of stage I-IIIB and pathologically verified residual cancer cells (no pathological complete response) after neoadjuvant chemotherapy underwent adjuvant treatment with gemcitabine plus cisplatin combined with regional hyperthermia [42]. For quality assurance, feasibility, efficacy, and toxicity of all treated patients were analyzed. Outcome was evaluated for the entire group of patients as well as for the subgroups of patients with or without lymph node involvement at baseline (cN0/cN+). From August 2012 to January 2019, this treatment was offered to 53 patients as part of routine care. The median follow-up was 38 months. Most patients (64.2%) had cT2 tumors at baseline. Twenty-four patients (45%) were clinically node positive as evaluated by sonography. Thirty-nine patients (74%) had grade 3, and 14 patients (26%) had grade 2 tumors. Forty-one patients (76%) showed a regression grade 1 according to Sinn. Patients received a median of six treatment cycles of gemcitabine and cisplatin (range 1-6) combined with 12 applications of regional hyperthermia (median 12, range 2-12). Disease-free survival (DFS) at 3 years was 57.5%. In patients with no lymph node involvement at baseline (cN0), DFS at 3 years was significantly higher than in initially node-positive (cN+) patients (80 vs. 31%; P=0.001). Overall survival (OS) at 3 years was 81.6%. In patients with no lymph node involvement at baseline (cN0), OS at 3 years was significantly higher than in node-positive (cN+) patients (93 vs. 70.4%; P=0.02). Overall, grade 3/4 toxicities were leukopenia (38%), thrombocytopenia (4%), and anemia (4%).

In conclusion of these results, after standard neoadjuvant chemotherapy containing anthracycline plus cyclophosphamide followed by taxanes, the addition of adjuvant gemcitabine plus cisplatin in combination with regional hyperthermia was safe and effective in TNBC patients with non-pCR.

3.2.7. Cervical Cancer

For cervical cancer recurrences following radiochemotherapy, the use of simultaneous application of weekly 50 mg/m² cisplatin (CDDP) and regional hyperthermia (RHT) resulted in a 50% response rate while the response rate was expected to be about 15% without regional hyperthermia [43, 44].

3.2.8. Pedriatic Cancer

Although the survival of children and adolescents with malignant germ-cell tumors has improved greatly in recent years, the outcome remains poor for those with **refractory or recurrent malignant germ-cell tumors.** A prospective study aimed to determine whether objective tumor response could be achieved in patients with refractory or recurrent malignant germ-cell tumors with chemotherapy combined with-regional deep hyperthermia as salvage treatment. In this controlled trial, patients with refractory or recurrent non-testicular malignant germ-cell tumors after standard cisplatin-based chemotherapy were treated prospectively with platin-etoposide-ifosfamide (PEI) chemotherapy (cisplatin 40 mg/m², on days 1 and 4; etoposide 100 mg/m², on days 1-4; and ifosfamide 1800 mg/m², on days 1-4) plus simultaneous 1-hour regional deep hyperthermia (41-43°C) on days 1 and 4. Patients received three to four treatment courses at 21-day intervals until residual tumor resection was possible; they subsequently received one or two additional courses of PEI-regional deep hyperthermia. Local radiotherapy was given for incompletely resected tumors. Chemotherapy and hyperthermia toxic effects were assessed using WHO grading. The primary endpoint was the proportion of patients who had an objective response as assessed with RECIST version 1.0 guidelines. Secondary endpoints were the event-free survival and overall survival after 5 years. The study (Hyper-PEI protocol) was registered at the German Cancer Society (45). 44 patients aged 7 months to 21 years (median 2 years 7 months) with refractory or recurrent malignant germ-cell tumors (nine patients with poor response, 23 patients with first relapse, 12 patients with multiple relapses) were included in this study. We identified 34 yolk sac tumours, eight embryonal carcinomas, one choriocarcinoma, and one dysgerminoma by histology analysis. Of the 35 patients who had sufficient clinical and radiographical data available for response assessment, 30 (86%) had an objective response to treatment (16 patients had complete remission and 14 had partial remission). 5-year event-free survival was 62% (95% CI, 45-75), and 5-year overall survival was 72% (95% CI, 55-83). The median follow-up of surviving patients was 82 months (range 9-195). WHO grade 3-4 neutropenia and thrombocytopenia occurred in all 181 chemotherapy cycles. Neutropenic fever, which required intercurrent hospital admission, was noted in 29 (66%) of 44 patients after 53 (29%) of 181 courses. Five patients experienced treatment-related grade-3 acute renal toxic effects

In summary, the multimodal strategy integrating salvage chemotherapy with regional hyperthermia and tumor resection with or without radiation can successfully treat children and adolescents with refractory or recurrent malignant non-testicular germ-cell tumors. The long-term prognosis of patients with poor response or after first relapse was almost like those receiving first-line treatment. The study offers a standardized treatment option for this subgroup of pediatric patients. Moreover, the well performed study confirmed the feasibility and safety of regional hyperthermia in the combination with standard chemotherapy and warrants further investigation in other solid pediatric tumors.

3.2.9. References

1. Lindner LH, Issels RD. Stellenwert der Hyperthermie im Rahmen der medikamentösen Tumortherapie. Der Onkologe 2010;16:1063-71.

2. Cihoric N, Tsikkinis A, van Rhoon G, et al. Hyperthermia-related clinical trials on cancer treatment within the ClinicalTrials.gov registry. Int J Hyperthermia 2015; 31:609-14.

3. Fujimoto S, Takahashi M, Mutou T, et al. Improved mortality rate of gastric carcinoma patients with peritoneal carcinomatosis treated with intraperitoneal hyperthermic chemoperfusion combined with surgery. Cancer 1997;79:884-91.

4. Loggie BW, Fleming RA, McQuellon RP, Russell GB, Geisinger KR, Levine EA. Prospective trial for the treatment of malignant peritoneal mesothelioma. Am Surg. 2001;67:999-1003.

5. Helm CW, Randall-Whitis L, Martin 3rd RS, et al. Hyperthermic intraperitoneal chemotherapy in conjunction with surgery for the treatment of recurrent ovarian carcinoma. Gynecol Oncol 2007;105:90-6.

6. Sugarbaker PH, Chang D. Results of treatment of 385 patients with peritoneal surface spread of appendiceal malignancy. Ann Surg Oncol 1999;6:727 31.

7. Verwaal VJ, van Ruth S, de Bree E, et al. Randomized trial of cytoreduction and hyperthermic intraperitoneal chemotherapy versus systemic chemotherapy and palliative surgery in patients with peritoneal carcinomatosis of colorectal cancer. J Clin Oncol 2003;21:3737-43.

8. Spilotis J. Hyperthermic intraperitoneal chemotherapy in ovarian cancer: Qui Bono? Ann Transl Med 2020; 8:1708.

9. Van Driel WJ, Koole SN, Skirska K, et al. Hyperthermic intraperitoneal chemotherapy in ovarian cancer. N Engl J Med 2018;378:230-240.

10. Souadka A, Essangri H, Anass Majbar M, et al. Hyperthermic intraperitoneal chemotherapy and cytoreductive surgery in ovarian cancer: An umbrella review of meta-analyses. Front Oncol 2022;12:809773.

11. Woldu SL, Bagrodia A, Lotan Y. Guideline of guidelines: non-muscle-invasive bladder cancer. BJU Int 2017; 119:371-80.

12. Angulo JC, Álvarez-Ossorio JL, Domínguez-Escrig JL, et al. Hyperthermic mitomycin C in intermediate-risk non-muscle-invasive bladder cancer: Results of the HIVEC-1 trial. Eur Urol Oncol 2023;6:58-66.

13. Tan WS, Steinberg G, Witjes JA, et al. Intermediate-risk Non-muscle-invasive bladder cancer: Updated consensus definition and management recommendations from the International Bladder Cancer Group. Eur Urol Oncol 2022;5:505-16.

14. Colombo R, da Pozzo LF, Salonia A et al. Multicentric study comparing intravesical chemotherapy alone and with local microwave hyperthermia for prophylaxis of recurrence of superficial transitional cell carcinoma. J Clin Oncol 2003;21:4270-6.

15. Colombo R, Salonia A, Leib Z, Pavone-Macaluso M, Engelstein D. Long-term outcomes of a randomized controlled trial comparing thermochemotherapy with mitomycin-C alone as adjuvant treatment for non-muscle-invasive bladder cancer (NMIBC). BJU Int 2011; 107:912-8.

16. Arends TJH, Nativ O, Maffezzini M, De Cobelli O, Van Der Heijden AG, Witjes JA. Results of the first randomized controlled trial comparing intravesical radiofrequency induced chemohyperthermia with mitomycin-C vs. BCG for adjuvant treatment of patients with intermediate-and high-risk non-muscle invasive bladder cancer. Eur Urol 2016;69:1046-52.

17. Tan WS, Panchal A, Buckley L, et al. Radiofrequency-induced thermo-chemotherapy effect versus a second course of *Bacillus Calmette-Guérin* or institutional standard in patients with recurrence of non-muscle-invasive bladder cancer following induction or maintenance *Bacillus Calmette-Guérin* therapy (HYMN): A phase III, open-label, randomised controlled trial. Eur Urol 2019; 75:63-71.

18. Carter DL, MacFall JR, Clegg ST, et al. Magnetic resonance thermometry during hyperthermia for human high-grade sarcoma. Int J Radiat Oncol Biol Phys 1998; 40:815-22.

19. Bertsch F, Mattner J, Stheling MK, et al. Non-invasive temperature mapping using MRI: comparison of two methods based on chemical shift and T1-relaxation. Magn Reson Imaging 1998;16:393-404.

20. Peller M, Löffler R, Baur A, et al. MRI-controlled regional hyperthermia. Radiologe 1999;39:756-763.

21. Gellermann J, Wlodarczyk W, Hildebrandt B, et al. Noninvasive Magnetic Resonance Thermography of Recurrent rectal carcinoma in a 1.5 Tesla hybrid system. Cancer Res 2005;65:5872-80.

22. Imman BA, Stauffer PR, Craciunescu OA, Maccarini PF, Dewhirst MW, Vujaskovic Z. A pilot clinical trial of intravesical mitomycin-C and external deep pelvic hyperthermia for non-muscle-invasive bladder cancer. Int J Hyperthermia 2014;30:171-5.

23. Wittlinger M, Rödel CM, Weiss C, et al. Quadrimodal treatment of high-risk T1 and T2 bladder cancer: transurethral tumor resection followed by concurrent radiochemotherapy and regional deep hyperthermia. Radiother Oncol 2009;93:358-63.

24. Geijsen ED, de Reijke TM, Koning CC, et al. Combining mitomycin C and regional 70 MHz hyperthermia in patients with nonmuscle invasive bladder cancer: A Pilot Study. J Urol 2015;194:1202-8.

25. Issels RD, Lindner LH, Verweij J, et al. Neo-adjuvant chemotherapy alone or with regional hyperthermia for localised high-risk soft-tissue sarcoma: a randomised phase 3 multicentre study. Lancet Oncol 2010;11:561-70.

26. Issels RD, Lindner LH, Verweij J, et al. Effect of neoadjuvant chemotherapy plus regional hyperthermia on long-term outcomes among patients with localized high-risk soft tissue sarcoma: The EORTC 62961-ESHO 95 Randomized Clinical Trial. JAMA Oncol 2018;4:483-92.

27. Lindner LH, Blay J-Y, Eggermont AMM, Issels RD. Perioperative chemotherapy and regional hyperthermia for high-risk adult-type soft tissue sarcomas. Eur J Cancer 2021;147:164-9.

28. Fiegl M, Schlemmer M, Wendtner C-M, Abdel-Rahman S, Fahn W, Issels RD. Ifosfamide, carboplatin and etoposide (ICE) as second-line regimen alone and in combination with regional hyperthermia is active in chemo-pre-treated advanced soft tissue sarcoma of adults. Int J Hyperthermia Abstract 2004.

29. Nickenig C, Buecklein V, Lindner LH, et al. Ifosfamide, carboplatin, and etoposide (ICE) in combination with regional hyperthermia (RHT) in chemotherapy-pretreated nonresponders with locally advanced high-risk soft tissue sarcoma (HR-STS). J Clin Oncol Abstract 2009.

30. Westermann AM, Wiedemann GJ, Jager E, et al. A Systemic Hyperthermia Oncologic Working Group trial. Ifosfamide, carboplatin, and etoposide combined with 41.8 degrees C whole-body hyperthermia for metastatic soft tissue sarcoma. Oncology 2003;64:312-21.

31. Hildebrandt B, Hegewisch-Becker S, Kerner T, et al. Current status of radiant whole-body hyperthermia at temperatures >41.5°C and practical guidelines for the treatment of adults. The German "Interdisciplinary Working Group of Hyperthermia". Int J Hyperthermia 2005:21:169-83.

32. Atanackovic D, Nierhaus A, Neumeier M, Hossfeld DK, Hegewisch-Becker S. 41.8 degrees C whole body hyperthermia as an adjunct to chemotherapy induces prolonged T cell activation in patients with various malignant diseases. Cancer Immunol Immunother 2002;51: 603-13.

33. Burd R, Dziedzic TS, Xu Y, Caligiuri MA, Subjeck JR, Repasky EA. Tumor cell apoptosis, lymphocyte recruitment and tumor vascular changes are induced by low temperature, long duration (fever-like) whole body hyperthermia. J Cell Physiol 1998;177:137-47.

34. Chen Q, Fisher DT, Clancy KA, et al. Fever-range thermal stress promotes lymphocyte trafficking across

high endothelial venules via an interleukin 6 trans-signaling mechanism. Nat Immunol 2006;7:1299-308.

35. Kraybill WG, Olenki T, Evans SS, et al. A phase I study of fever-range whole body hyperthermia (FR-WBH) in patients with advanced solid tumours: correlation with mouse models. Int J Hyperthermia 2002;18:253-66.

36. Kleef R, Nagy R, Baierl A, Bacher V, et al. Low-dose ipilimumab plus nivolumab combined with IL-2 and hyperthermia in cancer patients with advanced disease: exploratory findings of a case series of 131 stage IV cancers – a retrospective study of a single institution. Cancer Immunol Immunother 2021;70:1393-1403.

37. Bücklein V, Limmroth C, Kampmann E, et al. Ifosfamide, Carboplatin, and Etoposide (ICE) in combination with regional hyperthermia as salvage therapy in patients with locally advanced nonmetastatic and metastatic soft-tissue sarcoma. Sarcoma 2020;6901678.

38. Koops HS, Vaglini M, Suciu S, et al. Prophylactic isolated limb perfusion for localized, high-risk limb melanoma: results of a multicenter randomized phase III trial. J Clin Oncol 1998;16:2906-12.

39. Eggermont AM, de Wil JH, ten Hagen TL. Current uses of isolated limb perfusion in the clinic and a model system for new strategies. Lancet Oncol 2003;4:429-37.

40. Tschoep-Lechner KE, Milani V, Berger F, et al. Gemcitabine and cisplatin combined with regional hyperthermia as second-line treatment in patients with gemcitabine-refractory advanced pancreatic cancer. Int J Hyperthermia 2013;29:8-16.

41. Issels RD, Boeck S, Pelzer U, et al. Regional hyperthermia with cisplatin added to gemcitabine versus gemcitabine in patients with resected pancreatic ductal adenocarcinoma: The HEAT randomised clinical trial. Eur J Cancer 2023;181:155-165.

42. Stoetzer O, Di Gioia D, Issels RD, et al. Post-neoadjuvant gemcitabine and cisplatin with regional hyperthermia for patients with triple-negative breast cancer and non-pcr after neoadjuvant chemotherapy: A single-institute experience. Breast Care (Basel) 2021;16:173-180.

43. Rietbroek RC, Schilthuis MS, Bakker PJ, et al. Phase II trial of weekly locoregional hyperthermia and cisplatin in patients with a previously irradiated recurrent carcinoma of the uterine cervix. Cancer 1997;79:935-43.

44. De Wit R, van der Zee J, van der Burg ME, et al. A phase I/II study of combined weekly systemic cisplatin and locoregional hyperthermia in patients with previously irradiated recurrent carcinoma of the uterine cervix. Br J Cancer 1999:80:1387-1391.

45. Wessalowski R, Schneider DT, Mils O, et al. Regional deep hyperthermia for salvage treatment of children and adolescents with refractory or recurrent non-testicular malignant germ-cell tumours: an open-label, non-randomised, single-institution, phase 2 study. Lancet Oncol 2013;14:843-52.

3.3. Radiotherapy and Hyperthermia

The majority of the published randomized data evaluated the additional beneficial effects of local and regional hyperthermia in combination with radiotherapy. It has been shown in several tumor entities and different treatment schedules that additional heating with one or two sessions per week before or after the radiation fraction is able to improve clinical endpoints, including response, local control, and even overall survival rates. In these trials, late side effects were not usually increased by additional hyperthermia, which makes local or regional hyperthermia treatments attractive as radiosensitizer for the radiotherapist. A short overview summarizing published results of the beneficial effects of hyperthermia combined with radiotherapy has been provided below.

3.3.1. Breast Cancer

A total of six randomized trials analyzed the effects of combined thermoradiotherapy in breast cancer patients. Five of them were started between 1988 and 1991 by the UK Medical Research Council, the European Society of Hyperthermic Oncology (ESHO), the Dutch Hyperthermia Group, and the Princess Margaret Hospital/Ontario Cancer Institute [1]. Patients were eligible if they had advanced primary or recurrent breast cancer, and local radiotherapy was indicated in preference to surgery. The primary endpoint of all trials was local complete response. Slow recruitment led to a decision to collaborate and combine the trial results in one meta-analysis, and report them in one publication. A total of 306 patients were analyzed: 44% (135/306) received radiotherapy alone, and 56% (171/306) received combined treatment. The biologically effective radiation dose ranged between 40 and 70 Gy, the single fraction dose between 1.8 and 4 Gy, and the overall treatment time between 2 and 5 weeks. In the five trials, heat was applied utilizing different devices for superficial hyperthermia. Depending on the protocol, 2-8 hyperthermia treatments were scheduled during the radiation course. The duration of hyperthermia ranged between 45 and 70 minutes, and the prescribed target temperature in the tumor area was 42.5-43°C. The overall complete remission rate (n=306) for radiotherapy alone was 41%, and for the combined treatment 59% (P<0.001). The greatest effect was observed in patients with recurrent lesions in previously irradiated areas, where further irradiation was limited to low doses. Of the patients who received a complete remission, 17% received combined treatment, and 31% of the radiotherapy only patients had a local relapse during follow-up (P=0.007). The majority of the patients (227/306) showed progression of disease outside the treatment area during follow-up. The authors discussed this finding as evidence that overall survival was not improved by additional hyperthermia despite a significantly better local control. Hyperthermia was well tolerated and did not add to either the clinically relevant acute or long-term toxicity over irradiation alone, even in those patients who had received prior radiotherapy.

The authors concluded that the combined analysis of the five trials demonstrated the efficacy of hyperthermia as an adjunct to radiotherapy for the treatment of recurrent breast cancer.

The sixth trial evaluating the role of hyperthermia in the treatment of breast cancer was published in 2005 by the Radiation Department of the Duke University, North Carolina [2]. A total of 108 patients with superficially located tumors with different origins were analyzed in detail. The patients received either radiation alone (n=52) or radiation combined with superficial hyperthermia (n=56). Of the patients who received radiation alone, 63% (33/52) had breast cancer or chest wall recurrences after a history of breast cancer, 12% (6/52) had head and neck cancer, 12% (6/52) had malignant melanoma, and 13% (7/52) had other tumor histologies. In the combined group the distribution was 66% (37/56), 14% (8/56), 9% (5/56), and 11% (6/56), respectively. A separate analysis for the breast cancer patients only was not performed. Among patients in both arms, the median radiation dose, if prior radiation had been given, was 41 Gy (range, 18 to 66 Gy) and the median radiation dose, if no prior radiation had been given, was 60 Gy (range, 24 to 70 Gy). Patients were randomly assigned to receive no further hyperthermia (no-HT arm) or additional hyperthermia (HT arm) throughout the course of radiation, delivered twice a week for a maximum of 10 treatments, 1 to 2 hours in length, separated by at least 48 hours. Microwave spiral strip applicators, operating at 433 MHz, were used for external heating. Temperature was measured invasively. Maximally allowed temperatures in the adjacent normal tissue and tumor tissue were 43°C and 50°C, respectively. The complete remission rate in the HT arm was 66%; the CR rate in the no-HT arm was 42% (P=0.02). There was no significant difference in the proportion of patients in each arm who received additional systemic therapy. The improved local response in the high-dose arm resulted in a significant difference in duration of local control between the two arms (P=0.02). The high-dose arm had 48% local control at death or last follow-up versus 25% in the no-HT arm. The improvement in local control was most pronounced for patients who were previously irradiated; 15 of 22 patients in the HT arm (68%) had a complete remission versus four of 17 patients in the no-HT arm (24%). Overall survival was not significantly different between the two groups.

3.3.2. Rectal Cancer

A systematic Cochrane review analyzed all available randomized data on concomitant hyperthermia and radiation for the treatment of locally advanced rectal cancer [3]. Six randomized trials published between 1990 and 2000 were identified [4-9]. Four were single center [4-7] and two [8, 9] were multicenter trials. A total of 520 patients were treated, 258 in the radiotherapy only arm (RT) and 262 in the radiotherapy-hyperthermia arm (RHT). Four studies (424 patients) reported overall survival (OS) rates [4-8]. After 2 years, OS was significantly better in the RHT group (P=0.001), but this difference disappeared after a longer period. All but one studies reported complete remission rates [4, 5, 7-9]. A significantly higher complete remission rate was observed in the RHT group (P=0.01). Four studies reported on acute toxicity [5, 7-9]. Two of them showed no difference [5, 8] and the others [7, 9] only a slight increase between the RT and the RHT group. Late toxicity data were reported by van der Zee et al. only [8].

Berdov et al. [5] randomized 115 primary T4N0M0 rectal cancer patients to receive either preoperative RT (n=59) or RHT (n=56). The radiotherapy given in both study arms consisted of 40 Gy in 10 fractions given 3 times a week; local hyperthermia was applied 10 minutes before radiotherapy with target temperatures of 42-43°C over 60 minutes, 4-5 times during the radiation course. Pathologic complete tumor responses were obtained in 16.1% in the thermoradiotherapy group versus 1.7% in the radiotherapy alone group (P<0.05). Acute toxicity data were the same in both groups. The 2, 3 4 and year overall survival data were 48.1, 30.3, 25.0 and 21.4%. in the thermoradiotherapy group and 16.9, 15.0, 11.8 and 11.8% in the radiotherapy alone group (P<0.05).

Berdov et al. [4] randomized, in an additional trial, 93 patients (RT: n=45; RHT: n=48) with locally advanced (T2-4, N0-X, M0-1) rectal cancer. All patients got adjuvant chemotherapy with 5-FU. Total doses of 40 Gy in 10 fractions 3 times a week were given in the first part of treatment, with hyperthermia from the 3rd to 7th fraction. After a break of 4 weeks hyperfractionated daily RT of 1 Gy and 1.5 Gy with 4-hour interval was applied for a total of 30-40 Gy. Thus, total doses of 70-80 Gy were given. Response rates are reported after 40 Gy and after 70-80 Gy. Complete tumor responses were reported in 8 (17%) and 15 (31%) patients respectively in the RHT group versus 0 and 3 patients (7%) in the RT arm. Partial responses were seen in 36 (75%) and 33 (69%) patients after 40 and 70-80 Gy in the RHT arm and in 10 (22%) and 22 (49%) patients in the RT arm. 2- and 3-year OS in the non-metastasized patients were 36 and 17% in the RHT group versus 20 and 8% in the RT alone group (P=0.072). Local recurrence-free survival was better in the RHT group than in the RT alone group (P=0.041). No data on toxicity are given.

Kakehi et al. [6] reported on 14 patients randomized to receive either preoperative RT or RHT. Five patients got 40 Gy in 20 fractions of 2 Gy; nine patients got the same radiotherapy with a total of 10 hyperthermia sessions twice weekly thereafter, with intracavitary temperatures above 42°C lasting for 40-50 minutes. Partial responses were reported in all patients (100%) in the RHT group versus 20% (1/5) in the control group. No data on OS or acute and late toxicity are given.

Trotter et al. [7] reported on 73 patients; 9 of these had primary non-resectable and 64 recurrent rectal cancer. Twenty-three had metastasized at the time of randomization. They were randomized to receive either preoperative RT or RHT. The radiotherapy alone consisted of 50 Gy in 1.8 Gy daily fractions over a period of 6 weeks. In the RHT arm, radiation consisted of 36-40 Gy in 1.5 Gy daily fractions given in a 5-6-week period. Hyperthermia was performed on two or more days per week, 2 or 3 times, lasting 10 minutes with a 30-minute interval, directly before radiation. The median number of hyperthermia treatments was 26 (range, 4-52). The median dose in the combined arm was 42.75 Gy. Two patients in both arms had a pathological complete response. There was no significant difference in overall survival. Acute grade 3-4 toxicity was slightly higher in the RHT arm.

Van der Zee et al. [8] randomized 143 patients with primary or recurrent rectal cancer. The radiation dose was 46-50 Gy in 1.8-2.3 Gy daily fractions, followed, if possible, by a boost of 10-24 Gy to the tumor mass. Regional hyperthermia was prescribed once weekly, 1-4 hours after radiotherapy, lasting 60-90 minutes after reaching 42°C, for a total of five treatments. No significant differences in complete response and overall survival rates were found, although there was a trend to better results for the combined arm. Acute grade 3-4 toxicity did not differ between the two groups. Late toxicity was not significantly enhanced by the addition of hyperthermia.

You et al. [9] randomized 82 patients with rectal cancer preoperatively. The radiotherapy alone group got 30 Gy in 8 fractions of 3.75 Gy, twice a week, or 40 Gy in 2 Gy daily fractions given five times a week. The RHT group got the same radiation, either 30 or 40 Gy with endocavitary hyperthermia. The hyperthermia was applied 30 minutes after radiotherapy twice weekly, a total of 6-8 times during 5 minutes. The temperature reached was 45-50°C at the tumor surface. The pathological CR rate was 22.7% vs. 5.3% in favor of the combined treatment arm (P<0.05). Overall survival data are hard to report because nine patients (11%) had metastases at the time of randomization and not all patients got surgery after the given preoperative treatment. Acute toxicity was seen in 14% of the combined treatment arm versus 8% in the radiotherapy alone arm.

The analyzed trials and the comprehensive meta-analysis once more support the additional use of hyperthermia as a radiosensitizer. Of course, data quality is limited due to low patient numbers and selection biases of the analyzed trials. Therefore, the authors of the Cochrane review concluded that further studies are needed to compare thermo-radiation versus chemoradiation versus chemo-radiation combined with hyperthermia in well selected and conducted and quality controlled randomized clinical trials [3].

3.3.3. Cervical Carcinoma

Seven randomized trials evaluated the role of combined radiotherapy and hyperthermia in the treatment of locally advanced cervical cancer [10-15, 22].

The Dutch Deep Hyperthermia Trial [8, 12] compared radiotherapy with combined radiotherapy and regional hyperthermia in 114 women with locally advanced cervical carcinoma (FIGO stages IIB-IVA). Radiotherapy was applied to a median total dose of 68 Gy. Hyperthermia was administered once weekly. The primary end point was local control. Secondary end points were overall survival and late toxicity. After 12 years of follow-up, local control remained better in the combined group (37% vs. 56%; P=0.01). Furthermore, overall survival was better (20% vs. 37%; P=0.03). Late toxicities were similar in both groups. The authors concluded that for locally advanced cervical cancer the addition of regional hyperthermia to standard radiotherapy resulted in long-term significant improvement in local control and overall survival without increasing late toxicity, and therefore, this combined treatment should at least be considered for patients who are unfit to receive chemotherapy. Furthermore, the working group analyzed the intraluminally measured temperature at the tumor site and found significant better tumor control and survival rates for higher temperature values. The authors concluded that these results confirm the additional benefit of deep regional hyperthermia in combination with combined radiotherapy [21].

Harima et al. [13] investigated the role of thermo-radiotherapy in forty patients with FIGO Stage IIIB cervical carcinoma. Patients were treated with external beam irradiation to the pelvis, combined with Iridium-192 high-dose-rate intracavitary brachytherapy. The patients were randomly assigned to receive either radiotherapy alone (n=20) or thermoradiotherapy (n=20). The primary endpoint of this study was local complete response and survival. A complete response was achieved in 50% (10/20) in the radiotherapy group versus 80% (16/20) in the combined group (P=0.048). Three-year overall survival (58.2 and 63.6%) and disease-free survival (48.1 and 45%) of the patients in the hyperthermia group were better than those of the patients treated with radiotherapy alone, but these differences were not significant. The 3-year local relapse-free survival of the patients who were treated with hyperthermia was significantly better than that of the patients treated with radiotherapy (79.7% vs. 48.5%; P=0.048). The authors summarized that combined radiotherapy and hyperthermia was well tolerated and did not significantly add to either the relevant clinical acute or long-term toxicity over radiation alone, and resulted in a better treatment response and 3-year local relapse-free survival rate than RT for patients with FIGO Stage IIIB cervical carcinoma.

Datta et al. [11] reported on improved complete remission, pelvic control, and overall survival rates in 64 patients with cervical cancer (FIGO IIIB) in favor of the combined therapy group with radiation and hyperthermia.

Chen et al. [10] randomly compared radiation with and without hyperthermia in 120 patients with FIGO IIB-IIIB disease. They found a significantly better complete response rate in favor of the combined treatment approach.

Sharma et al. [14] reported on a better pelvic control (70% vs. 50%) in a randomized trial with a total of 50 patients (FIGO stages II-III).

A multi-institutional randomized trial included a total of 110 patients with locally advanced carcinoma of the uterine cervix who received radiotherapy with or without hyperthermia [15]. Each patient received external beam radiation therapy and brachytherapy, and a minimum of five hyperthermia sessions once weekly. At a median follow-up period of 42 months the overall survival rate at 3 years was 73.2%, and the local control rate was 68.5%. There were no significant differences between the patients treated with or without hyperthermia. There was no significant difference in the late toxicity observed in the two arms. This study failed to show any benefit from the addition of hyperthermia to radiotherapy in the treatment of locally advanced carcinoma of the uterine cervix. A probable explanation for this is that an adequate hyperthermia dose was applied to only part of the tumor [16].

In 2016, Lutgens et al. reported on the randomized RADCHOC trial [32]. This multicenter study tried to establish if radiotherapy combined with hyperthermia (RT-HT group) should be preferred over cisplatin-based chemoradiation (RT-CT group) in bulky and/or FIGO-stage ≥III. The primary endpoint was event-free survival (EFS). Because of slow recruitment, the trial was closed prematurely: 87 of 376 planned patients were enrolled between 2003 and 2009. The median follow-up was 7.1 years. The cumulative incidence of any event was 33% in the RT-CT group and 35% in the RT-HT group (n.s.). Pelvic progression-free survival and overall survival rates were similar, as well. Additionally no differences were described for grade ≥3 radiation related late toxicity. Based on the available data, the authors concluded that the outcomes were comparable in both arms.

3.3.4. Further Results

Further significant benefits for the additional use of hyperthermia in combination with standard radiotherapy have been reported for some other tumor entities.

Interstitial hyperthermia improved local control and overall survival in the treatment of glioblastoma multiforme [17] and superficial hyperthermia improved local control using combined treatment for malignant melanoma [18]. Additionally hyperthermia improved local control in definitive treatment of head and neck cancer [19, 20, 23].

3.3.5. References

1. Vernon CC, Hand JW, Field SB, et al. Radiotherapy with or without hyperthermia in the treatment of superficial localized breast cancer: results from five randomized controlled trials. International Collaborative Hyperthermia Group. Int J Radiat Oncol Biol Phys 1996; 35:731-744.

2. Jones EL, Oleson JR, Prosnitz LR, et al. Randomized trial of hyperthermia and radiation for superficial tumors. J Clin Oncol 2005;23:3079-3085.

3. De Haas-Kock DF, Buijsen J, Pijls-Johannesma M, et al. Concomitant hyperthermia and radiation therapy for treating locally advanced rectal cancer. Cochrane Database Syst Rev 2009:CD006269.

4. Berdov BA, Kurpeshev OK, Mardinsky Yu S. Influence of Hyperthermia and Hyperglycemia on Efficiency Radiation Therapy for Oncological Patients. Russian Journal of Oncology 1996.

5. Berdov BA, Menteshashvili GZ. Thermoradiotherapy of patients with locally advanced carcinoma of the rectum. Int J Hyperthermia 1990;6:881-890.

6. Kakehi M, Ueda K, Mukojima T, et al. Multi-institutional clinical studies on hyperthermia combined with radiotherapy or chemotherapy in advanced cancer of deep-seated organs. Int J Hyperthermia 1990;6:719-740.

7. Trotter JM, Edis AJ, Blackwell JB, et al. Adjuvant VHF therapy in locally recurrent and primary unresectable rectal cancer. Australas Radiol 1996;40:298-305.

8. van der Zee J, Gonzalez Gonzalez D, van Rhoon GC, et al. Comparison of radiotherapy alone with radiotherapy plus hyperthermia in locally advanced pelvic tumours: a prospective, randomised, multicentre trial. Dutch Deep Hyperthermia Group. Lancet 2000;355:1119-1125.

9. You QS, Wang RZ, Suen GQ, et al. Combination preoperative radiation and endocavitary hyperthermia for rectal cancer: long-term results of 44 patients. Int J Hyperthermia 1993;9:19-24.

10. Chen HW J JF, Wei L. A randomized trial of hyper thermo-radiochemotherapy for uterine cervix cancer. Chin J Clin Oncol 1997;24:249-251.

11. Datta N.R. BAK, Kapoor H.K. Thermoradiotherapy in the management of carcinoma cervix (stage IIIB): A controlled clinical study. Indian Med Gaz 1987;121:68-71.

12. Franckena M, Stalpers LJ, Koper PC, et al. Long-term improvement in treatment outcome after radiotherapy and hyperthermia in locoregionally advanced cervix cancer: an update of the Dutch Deep Hyperthermia Trial. Int J Radiat Oncol Biol Phys 2008;70:1176-1182.

13. Harima Y, Nagata K, Harima K, et al. A randomized clinical trial of radiation therapy versus thermoradiotherapy in stage IIIB cervical carcinoma. Int J Hyperthermia 2001;17:97-105.

14. Sharma S PF, Sandhu AP, et al. A prospective randomized study of local hyperthermia as a supplement and radiosensitizer in the treatment of carcinoma of the cervix with radiotherapy. Endocuriether/Hyperthermia Oncol 1989;5:151-159.

15. Vasanthan A, Mitsumori M, Park JH, et al. Regional hyperthermia combined with radiotherapy for uterine cervical cancers: a multi-institutional prospective randomized trial of the international atomic energy agency. Int J Radiat Oncol Biol Phys 2005;61:145-153.

16. van der Zee J, van Rhoon GC, Wust P. In regard to Dr. Vasanthan et al. (Int J Radiat Oncol Biol Phys 2005;

61:145-153). Int J Radiat Oncol Biol Phys 2005;62:940-941.

17. Sneed PK, Stauffer PR, McDermott MW, et al. Survival benefit of hyperthermia in a prospective randomized trial of brachytherapy boost +/- hyperthermia for glioblastoma multiforme. Int J Radiat Oncol Biol Phys 1998;40:287-295.

18. Overgaard J, Gonzalez Gonzalez D, Hulshof MC, et al. Randomised trial of hyperthermia as adjuvant to radiotherapy for recurrent or metastatic malignant melanoma. European Society for Hyperthermic Oncology. Lancet 1995;345:540-543.

19. Datta NR, Bose AK, Kapoor HK, et al. Head and neck cancers: results of thermoradiotherapy versus radiotherapy. Int J Hyperthermia 1990;6:479-486.

20. Valdagni R, Amichetti M. Report of long-term follow-up in a randomized trial comparing radiation therapy and radiation therapy plus hyperthermia to metastatic lymph nodes in stage IV head and neck patients. Int J Radiat Oncol Biol Phys 1994;28:163-169.

21. Franckena M, Fatehi D, de Bruijne M, et al. Hyperthermia dose-effect relationship in 420 patients with cervical cancer treated with combined radiotherapy and hyperthermia. Eur J Cancer 2009;45:1969-78

22. Lutgens L, Koper P, Jobsen J et al. Radiation therapy combined with hyperthermia versus cisplatin for locally advanced cervical cancer: Results of the randomized RADCHOC trial. Radiother Oncol 2016;120:378-382.

23. Datta NR, Rogers S, Ordonez SG, et al. Hyperthermia and radiotherapy in the management of head and neck cancers: A systematic review and meta-analysis. Int J Hyperthermia 2016;32:31-40.

3.4. Radiochemotherapy and Hyperthermia

The concurrent use of radiotherapy, chemotherapy and local or regional hyperthermia techniques for the treatment of malignant diseases is under continuous development. In the last decade, the number of controlled trials addressing the combination of radiochemotherapy and heat significantly increased. These trials illustrate the radio- and chemosensitizing potential and the current limitations of additional hyperthermia in the framework of chemoradiation protocols.

3.4.1. Breast Cancer

Up to date, one randomized phase II trial [20] addressed the question of reirradiation and hyperthermia versus reirradiation and hyperthermia plus cisplatin-based chemotherapy for locally recurrent, non-resectable breast cancer in a previously irradiated chest wall area. From 2010 to 2019, 49 patients were randomized. Either 32 Gy was given in eight fractions of 4 Gy/4 weeks, two fractions per week, or 46 Gy in 23 fractions of 2 Gy, at five fractions per week. As part of the oncological standard treatment, hyperthermia was added once a week after radiotherapy. Additionally, patients in the experimental arm received four cycles of weekly cisplatin (40 mg/m²). Complete response rates were high and similar with 61% in both arms, partial response rates were 30% and 33%, respectively. One-year overall survival was 63% in the standard arm and 57% in the experimental arm with additional cisplatin. The one-year local progression-free interval was 82% in the standard arm and 88% in the experimental arm. Grade 3-4 early toxicity rates were 25% and 29%, similar as well. The authors concluded that the addition of cisplatin did not lead to a detectable further improvement of the very good results after combined radiotherapy and local hyperthermia in this small phase II trial.

3.4.2. Rectal Cancer

Between 1994 and 1999, 137 patients with locally advanced rectal carcinoma (≥uT3) were randomly treated by neoadjuvant radiochemotherapy with (50.4%) or without (49.6%) deep regional hyperthermia [1]. 5-fluorouracil (300-350 mg/m²) and leucovorin (50 mg) were administered on days 1 to 5 and 22 to 26. Deep regional hyperthermia was given once a week before radiotherapy (45 Gy with 1.8-Gy fractions for 5 weeks). Surgery followed 4-6 weeks after completion of neoadjuvant treatment. In an interim analysis in 2000, the response rate (complete and partial response rates) was significantly better (66% vs. 49%, $P<0.05$) for patients who received additional hyperthermia. The time to local recurrence was also better (28 vs. 20, $P<0.05$). Overall survival probability after 3 years follow-up was 89% vs. 80%, in favor of the hyperthermia group, but this difference was not statistically significant. At the time of the interim analysis local control was 93% in both arms after complete resection. Mature data for this trial were expected for 2005, but have not published to date. Despite the limitations in sample size and follow-up time, this trial provides some encouraging evidence of the effects of additional regional hyperthermia in com-

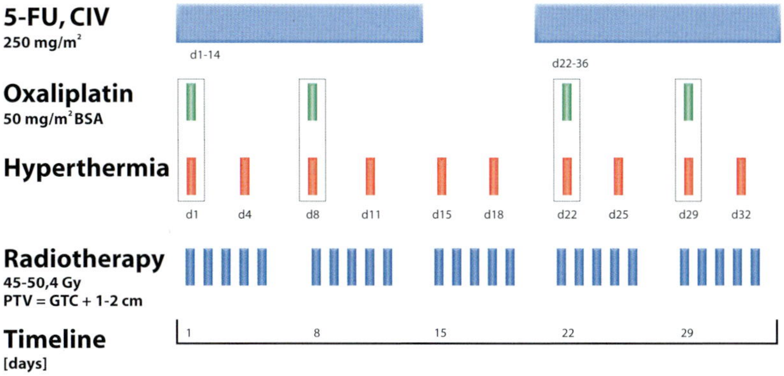

Figure 3.1: Flow chart of the HyRec trial [22]

bination with neoadjuvant radiochemotherapy in patients with locally advanced rectal cancer.

A Cochrane review summarized the existing evidence for the possible beneficial effects of additional hyperthermia in combination with radiotherapy [2]. A total of 520 patients from six randomized trials were analyzed. After 2 years, overall survival was significantly better in the hyperthermia group (P=0.001) compared to radiotherapy alone, but this difference disappeared after a longer period. Furthermore, a significantly higher pathologically complete remission rate (pCR) was observed in the hyperthermia group (P=0.01). Regarding acute toxicity no significant differences were observed by the addition of hyperthermia. Data on late toxicity was not available. The authors concluded that further studies are needed in well-selected and quality-controlled randomized trials.

Gani et al. [15] published a prospective phase II trial with 78 patients with locally advanced rectal cancer treated between 2012 and 2017. The patients received standard 5-fluorouracil-based neoadjuvant radiochemotherapy with 50.4 Gy in 28 fractions. Additionally, deep regional hyperthermia was applied twice weekly. The primary endpoint was pathological complete response. Median follow-up was 54 months. A pathological complete response (pCR) was reported in 14% of the patients, 50% had either a tumor regression grading of Dworak 4 (complete regression) or Dworak 3 (scattered tumor cells only). Three-year estimates for OS, DFS, LC and DC were 94%, 81%, 96% and 87%. Patients with higher hyperthermia-related cumulative temperatures showed stronger tumor regression.

Ott et al. [16] reported on a prospective multicenter trial (HyRec trial) for patients with locally advanced (LARC) or locally recurrent rectal cancer (LRRC). Between 2012 and 2018, 111 patients with UICC stage IIB-IV or any locally recurrent rectal cancer were included. Patients received radiotherapy (45-50 Gy/5 weeks) with concurrent 5-fluorouracil (5-FU)/capecitabine and oxaliplatin, and deep regional hyperthermia. Primary endpoints were the feasibility rate based on an analysis of dose-limiting toxicities and the pCR-rate. According to the protocol, the feasibility rates analyzed after19 and 59 treated patients were 90% (17/19) and 73% (43/59). Therefore, the protocol was judged as feasible. In the intention-to-treat population, the pCR rate was 19% (20/105; 90% confidence interval (CI) 13.0-26.5). In the per-protocol-analysis, complete tumor regression was seen in 28% (18/64) and 38% (3/8) of the patients with LARC and LRRC, respectively. The good remission rates were regarded as a real progress compared the results of the same regimen without hyperthermia. This prospective study offers a well-evaluated and safe curative regimen especially for patients with LRRC.

3.4.3. Cervical Carcinoma

The combination of external beam irradiation and brachytherapy and a concurrent cisplatin-based chemotherapy was established as a standard treatment for the locally advanced cervical cancer FIGO stage IIB-IVA during the past two decades. During that period, studies were initiated to test whether additional deep regional hyperthermia could further improve the oncological outcomes.

Westermann et al. reported on long-term survival data of a multicenter prospective trial for 68 patients with cervical cancer FIGO-stage IIB-IVA [17, 18]. Patients received a combination of radiotherapy (external beam radiotherapy and brachytherapy for a biologically effective dose of at least 86.7 Gy), four sessions of weekly locoregional hyperthermia, and concurrent chemotherapy (at least four courses of weekly cisplatin, 40 mg/m²). Median follow-up was 81 months. Five-year recurrence-free survival and overall survival rates were 58% and 66%, respectively. The authors concluded that the results were comparable to previous reports for this patient group in randomized trials.

A Polish phase III trial compared standard external beam radiochemotherapy (45-50 Gy) with a high-dose-rate brachytherapy boost with Ir-192 (four fractions with 7.5 Gy) alone or combined with interstitial hyperthermia (four treatments with 60 minutes, target temperature ≥42°C) in patients with locally advanced cervical cancer FIGO stage II-III [19]. Between 2006 and 2009, 224 consecutive patients were randomly assigned to the two treatment arms, 209 patients entered analysis. After a median follow-up of 45 months, an effect of hyperthermia was not detected for disease-free survival or for local control. Statistical differences were not observed for the distribution of early and late complications.

A randomized trial from Japan reported on 101 patients with cervical cancer FIGO IB-IVA, who received either cisplatin-based standard chemoradiotherapy with or without once weekly whole-pelvic hyperthermia [20]. Although not statistically significant, the 5-year overall, disease-free and local recurrence-free survival rates were better in the group with hyperthermia (78% vs. 65%, 71% vs. 61%, and 80% vs. 71%). Complete remission was significantly more likely to be achieved in patients with hyperthermia (88% vs. 78%, P=0.047). Hyperthermia caused no additional acute or long-term toxicity compared with CRT alone. An additional thermal dose parameter analysis revealed a better local relapse-free survival in both univariate and multivariate analyses for patients with a CEM43T90 >1 min (a thermal dose parameter) [21]. Disease-free survival and complete response rates showed a trend to better results in this group. Disease-free survival, local relapse-free survival and complete response rates for patients with a CEM43T90 >1 min were significantly better than those for patients with standard chemoradiation without hyperthermia (P=0.036, P=0.036, and P=0.048).

A Chinese randomized trial reported on 373 patients with cervical cancer FIGO stage IB-IV enrolled between 2009 and 2013 [22]. All patients received standard external beam irradiation with a high-dose-rate intracavitary brachytherapy boost and concurrent chemotherapy with 5-fluorouracil and cisplatin. In the experimental arm, regional hyperthermia was applied: total of 6 treatments, twice a week, target temperature in the vagina/rectum 40.5°C, session duration 60 minutes. Five-year overall survival was better with hyperthermia (82% vs. 72%, P=0.040). This was confirmed in a multivariate Cox regression analysis. The 5-year local relapse-free survival was also better (87% vs. 83%), but the difference was not significant. Early or late toxicity was not significantly different between the two groups.

Minnaar et al. showed preliminary data of an ongoing randomized trial for patients with locally advanced cervical cancer FIGO stage IIB-IIIB [23]. All patients received a standard definitive protocol with external beam irradiation and an Ir-192 brachytherapy boost with a total equivalent dose in 2 Gy fractions (for an alpha-beta ratio of 10) of 86 Gy. All participants were prescribed two doses of 80 mg/m² cisplatin, administered 21 days apart during external beam radiotherapy. The patients received two modulated electro-hyperthermia treatments per week. Disease recurrence at two and three years was significantly reduced in the hyperthermia group. There were no significant differences in late toxicity between the groups.

3.4.4. Anal Cancer

A Greek study group investigated the clinical benefit of the addition of intracavitary hyperthermia to a conventional radiochemotherapy schedule in patients with T2-T3N0M0 anal cancer [3]. Patients were randomly assigned to undergo chemotherapy with 5-fluorouracil (5-FU) and mitomycin-C combined with radiotherapy with or without intracavitary hyperthermia. A microwave applicator operating at 433 MHz inserted into the anal-rectal cavity was used. Patients in both arms received 1000 mg/m² per day of 5-FU on days 1-4 and days 28-31 plus 15 mg/m² mitomycin-C on day 1. Radiotherapy was administered with a dose of 41.4 Gy (1.8 Gy per fraction) plus a boost of 14 Gy (2 Gy per fraction). No severe morbidity was noted in the patients in either group. After a 5-year follow-up in the hyperthermia arm, 23 of 24 patients (95.8%) preserved their anorectal function and avoided permanent colostomy, whereas in the control arm, 17 of 25 (68.0%) had sphincter preservation.

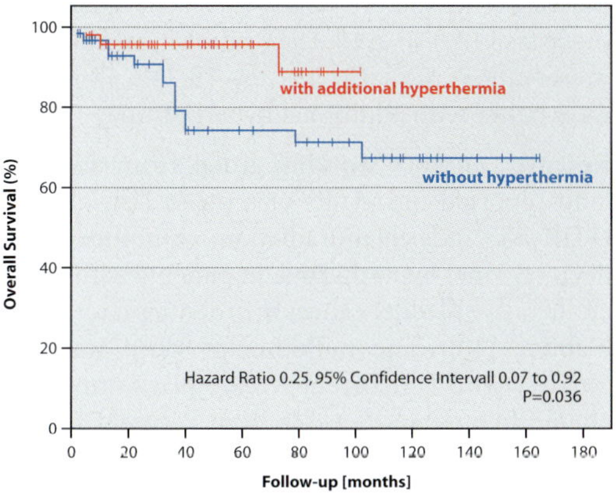

Figure 3.2: Overall survival rates after chemoradiation with and without deep regional hyperthermia for anal cancer [24].

Local recurrence-free survival time was significantly higher in the hyperthermia arm (P=0.01). No significant difference in overall survival was noted. This small randomized trial provided some information that the addition of intracavitary hyperthermia to the radiochemotherapy schedule may further improve relevant clinical endpoints; e.g., a higher preservation rate of anorectal function.

The prospective data of the randomized trial was confirmed by a retrospective analysis of 112 consecutive patients with anal cancer UICC stage I-IV treated between 2000 and 2015 [24]. All patients received chemoradiotherapy with 5-fluororuracil and mitomycin C. In case of insufficient tumor response 4-6 weeks after chemoradiotherapy, patients received an interstitial pulsed-dose-rate brachytherapy boost. Additionally, 50/112 patients received deep regional hyperthermia treatments. Median follow-up was 41 months. After five years follow-up, the patients with additional hyperthermia showed better overall survival (96% vs. 75%, P=0.045), disease-free survival (89% vs. 70%, P=0.027), local recurrence-free survival (98% vs. 79%, P=0.006), and colostomy-free survival rates (88% vs. 69%, P=0.016). Early toxicities grade 3-4 were comparable with the exception of hematotoxicity, which was higher in the group with additional hyperthermia (66% vs. 43%, P=0.032). Late side effects were similar with the exception of a higher perianal telangiectasia among the patients with hyperthermia (38% vs. 16%, P=0.009).

A randomized phase II trial comparing standard chemoradiation with and without additional deep regional hyperthermia (HyCAN trial) is in the terminal phase of patient recruitment. Further details on that trial may be found in Chapter 5.2 of this book.

3.4.5. Bladder Cancer

For decades, it has been a well-known fact that additional hyperthermia with 40-43°C combined with standard chemotherapy and/or radiotherapy may improve oncological outcomes such as local control, survival, and organ preservation rates in both superficial and muscle-invasive bladder cancer. This efficacy gain was not related to an increase of treatment related early or late toxicity rates, which makes hyperthermia an attractive radio- and chemosensitizer in the organ preserving treatment of bladder cancer [25].

The first randomized trial on the combination of external beam radiation with or without additional deep regional hyperthermia for the organ preserving treatment of muscle-invasive bladder cancer was published in 2000 [26]. From 1990 to 1996, 101 patients with T2-4N0-1 bladder cancer were included. External beam radiotherapy was applied conventionally fractionated with 66-70 Gy to the whole bladder, and 40 Gy to the regional pelvic lymph nodes. Hyperthermia was prescribed once weekly during the period of external radiotherapy, the intravesical target temperature was 42°C. The addition of heat to radiotherapy led to better complete response rates (73% vs. 51%, P=0.01). At the 3-year follow-up, the local control rate was 42% and 33% in favor of the hyperthermia group (P= n.s.), the overall survival rate was 28% vs. 22% (P=0.33), respectively. In summary, this trial confirmed the beneficial potential of additional hyperthermia in bladder cancer, but the improvement of the response rate did not translate into better local control or overall survival rates during follow-up.

In 2009, clinical data on the combination of standard chemoradiation and deep regional hyperthermia as bladder preserving treatment was published for the first time [27]. Forty-five patients with high-risk T1-2 bladder cancer were included and received an initial transurethral resection of the bladder tumor (iTUR-BT) followed by cisplatin-based chemoradiation (total dose 55-60 Gy, concurrent chemotherapy with 5-FU and cisplatin in the first and fifth irradiation week). Hyperthermia was given with 1-2 treatments per week and a total of 5-10 sessions during the radiotherapy series. After a median follow-up of 34 months, the complete response rate was 96%, this was histologically confirmed after an obligatory reevaluation transurethral resection (reTUR-BT) performed 4-6 weeks after the end of chemoradiation. Local recurrence-free survival was 85%, overall survival was 80%, disease-specific survival was 88%, metastasis-free survival was 89%, and the bladder-preserving rate was 96% (43/45) at 3 years. Analysis of risk factors for the first time revealed a better overall survival for patients who received ≥5 vs. <5 additive hyperthermia treatments.

Merten et al. summarized the long-term experience of chemoradiation without and combined with deep regional hyperthermia [28]. Between 1982 and 2016, 369 patients with pTa, pTis, pT1, and pT2 cN0-1 cM0 bladder cancer were treated with a multimodal treatment after initial TUR-BT. All patients received radiotherapy (RT) of the bladder and the regional lymph nodes. Concomitant chemoradiation was administered to 215/369 patients, chemoradiation combined with hyperthermia to 79/369, and radiotherapy alone was used in 75/369 patients. The median number of RHT treatments applied was 5 (range 1-10). At a median follow-up of 71 months, 5-year overall survival rates were 87% vs. 64% (P=0.0001) in favor of the patients with chemoradiation and additional hyperthermia compared to chemoradiation alone. Bladder preservation rates at 5 and 10 years were 96% vs. 82% and 96% vs. 78%, respectively. This was confirmed in the multivariate Cox regression analysis.

In the recent subgroup analysis from the same working group, 181 patients were analyzed who all received an iTUR-BT followed by or most effective chemoradiation schedule with 5-fluorouracil and cisplatin combined with (n=76) or without (n=105) additional deep regional hyperthermia [29]. In this collective, UICC category T3-4 was present in 19/181 patients (11%). Patient characteristics especially regarding UICC TNM stage were equally distributed in both arms. After a median follow-up of 75 months, 5-year overall survival (82.5% vs. 65.0%; P=0.015), 5-year disease-free survival (67.6% vs. 42.7%; P=0.003), local recurrence (26.3% vs. 46.7%; P=0.004), distant metastasis (4.0% vs. 19.0%; P=0.002), and bladder preservation rates (92.1% vs. 75.2%; P=0.004) were better with additional hyperthermia.

Recently, another working group from Switzerland reported on results of a phase II trial after iTUR-BT and chemoradiation combined with deep regional hyperthermia in patients with muscle-invasive bladder cancer in order to preserve the bladder [30]. The radiotherapy dose was 57-58.2 Gy with concurrent weekly platinum-based chemotherapy and weekly deep regional hyperthermia. Altogether 27 patients were included. The complete response rate was 93%. The 2-year cystectomy-free rate, PFS, LRFS and OS rates were 95%, 76%, 81% and 86%, respectively. The multimodal treatment was well tolerated with acute and late G3-4 toxicities of 10% and 13%, respectively. The authors concluded that the multimodal treatment with hyperthermia showed promising results with excellent local response and moderate toxicity.

3.4.6. Esophageal Carcinoma

From January 1988 to June 1992, Kitamura et al. [4] entered 66 patients with resectable squamous cell carcinoma of the thoracic esophagus in a prospective randomized trial. Thirty-two were treated with neoadjuvant radiofrequency wave local hyperthermia combined with radiochemotherapy, while the remaining 34 patients received radiochemotherapy alone. Radiation was applied with 2 Gy single fraction dose, five days per week, to a total dose of 30 Gy. Concurrent chemotherapy was delivered using bleomycin (5 mg i.v., two times per week, cumulative dose 30 mg), or cisplatin (40 mg/m^2 i.v., once per week, cumulative dose 120 mg/m^2). In the hyperthermia group, no viable cancer cells were found within the entire 5-mmwidth slices of the resected specimen in eight patients (25%) versus two (5.9%) in the control group ($P<0.05$). The cumulative 3-year overall survival rate was 50.4% and 24.2%, respectively (no P-value supplied). The authors concluded that the addition of hyperthermia to radiochemotherapy resulted in a better local control and an improved long-term survival when treating patients with advanced esophageal carcinoma.

A metaanalysis summarized the results of chemoradiation combined with regional hyperthermia for advanced esophageal cancer [31]. Nineteen randomized controlled trials with 1519 patients were analyzed. The metaanalysis revealed better overall survival rates, lower local recurrence and distant metastasis rates in favor of the patients with additional hyperthermia in comparison to the patients with chemoradiation and radiotherapy alone.

3.4.7. Further Fields of Research

The promising combination of concurrent radiochemotherapy and hyperthermia has already been explored in the framework of phase II and III trials for a number of additional malignancies; e.g. pancreatic cancer [9, 10], soft tissue sarcoma [11] and gallbladder and bile duct carcinoma [12, 13].

3.4.8. References

1. Rau BBT, Wust P, Schlag PM. Stellenwert der Hyperthermie für die chirurgische Onkologie. Viszeralchirurgie 2002;37:379-384.

2. De Haas-Kock DF, Buijsen J, Pijls-Johannesma M et al. Concomitant hyperthermia and radiation therapy for treating locally advanced rectal cancer. Cochrane Database Syst Rev 2009:CD006269.

3. Kouloulias V, Plataniotis G, Kouvaris J et al. Chemoradiotherapy combined with intracavitary hyperthermia for anal cancer: feasibility and long-term results from a phase II randomized trial. Am J Clin Oncol 2005;28:91-99.

4. Kitamura K, Kuwano H, Watanabe M et al. Prospective randomized study of hyperthermia combined with chemoradiotherapy for esophageal carcinoma. J Surg Oncol 1995;60:55-58.

5. Jones EL, Samulski TV, Dewhirst MW et al. A pilot Phase II trial of concurrent radiotherapy, chemotherapy, and hyperthermia for locally advanced cervical carcinoma. Cancer 2003;98:277-282.

6. Westermann AM, Jones EL, Schem BC et al. First results of triple-modality treatment combining radiotherapy, chemotherapy, and hyperthermia for the treatment of patients with stage IIB, III, and IVA cervical carcinoma. Cancer 2005;104:763-770.

7. Weiss C, Ott OJ, Wittlinger M et al. Treatment options for high-risk T1 bladder cancer: status quo and future perspectives of radiochemotherapy. Strahlenther Onkol 2008;184:443-449.

8. Ott OJ, Rodel C, Weiss C et al. Radiochemotherapy for Bladder Cancer. Clin Oncol (R Coll Radiol) 2009;21: 557-65.

9. Kouloulias VE, Nikita KS, Kouvaris JR, et al. Intraoperative hyperthermia and chemoradiotherapy for inoperable pancreatic carcinoma. Eur J Cancer Care (Engl) 2002;11:100-107.

10. Ohguri T, Imada H, Yahara K, et al. Concurrent chemoradiotherapy with gemcitabine plus regional hyperthermia for locally advanced pancreatic carcinoma: initial experience. Radiat Med 2008;26:587-596.

11. Ivanov SM, Tkachev SI, Bokhian B, et al. Thermoradiochemotherapy of inoperable soft-tissue sarcoma. Vopr Onkol 2005;51:350-354.

12. Kamisawa T, Tu Y, Ishiwata J, et al. Thermo-chemoradiotherapy for advanced gallbladder carcinoma. Hepatogastroenterol 2005;52:1005-1010.

13. Kamisawa T, Tu Y, Egawa N, et al. Thermo-chemoradiotherapy for advanced bile duct carcinoma. World J Gastroenterol 2005;11:4206-4209.

14. Schouten D, van Os R, Westermann AM, et al. A randomized phase-II study of reirradiation and hyperthermia versus reirradiation and hyperthermia plus chemotherapy for locally recurrent breast cancer in previously irradiated area. Acta Oncologica 2022;61:441-448.

15. Gani C et al. Deep regional hyperthermia with preoperative radiochemotherapy in locally advanced rectal cancer, a prospective phase II trial. Radiother Oncol 2021;159:155-6.

16. Ott OJ et al. Neoadjuvant chemoradiation combined with regional hyperthermia in locally advanced or recurrent rectal cancer. Cancers (Basel) 2021;13(6):1279.

17. Westermann AM, Jones EL, Schem BC, et al. First results of triple-modality treatment combining radiotherapy, chemotherapy, and hyperthermia for the treatment of patients with stage IIB, III, and IVA cervical carcinoma. Cancer 2005;104:763-70.

18. Westermann A, Mella O, van der Zee O, et al. Long-term survival data of triple modality treatment of stage IIB-III-IVA cervical cancer with the combination of radiotherapy, chemotherapy and hyperthermia – an update. Int J Hyperthermia 2012;28:549-553.

19. Zolciak-Siwinska A, Piotrkowicz N, Jonska-Gmyrek J, et al. HDR brachytherapy combined with interstitial hyperthermia in locallyadvanced cervical cancer patients initially treated with concomitant radiochemotherapy – a phase III study. Radiother Oncol 2013;109:194-199.

20. Harima Y, Ohguri T, Imada H, et al. A multicentre randomised clinical trial of chemoradiotherapy plus hyperthermia versus chemoradiotherapy alone in patients with locally advanced cervical cancer. Int J Hyperthermia 2016;32:801-808.

21. Ohguri T, Harima Y, Imada H, et al. Relationships between thermal dose parameters and the efficacy of definitive chemoradiotherapy plus regional hyperthermia in the treatment of locally advanced cervical cancer: data from a multicentre randomised clinical trial. Int J Hyperthermia 2018;34:461-8.

22. Wang Y, Hong W, Shaomin MS, et al. Outcomes for hyperthermia combined with concurrent radiochemotherapy for patients with cervical cancer. Int J Radiation Oncol Biol Phys 2020;107:499-511.

23. Minnaar CA, Maposa I, Kotzen JA, et al. Effects of modulated electro-hyperthermia (mEHT) on two and three year survival of locally advanced cervical cancer patients. Cancers (Basel) 2022;14:656.

24. Ott OJ, Schmidt M, Semrau S, et al. Chemoradiotherapy with and without deep regional hyperthermia for squamous cell carcinoma of the anus. Strahlenther Onkol 2019;195:607-614.

25. Ott OJ, Gaipl US, Lamrani A, et al. The Emerging evidence supporting integration of deep regional hyperthermia with chemoradiation in bladder cancer. Semin Radiat Oncol 2023;33:82-90.

26. van der Zee J, Gonzalez Gonzalez D, van Rhoon GC, et al. Comparison of radiotherapy alone with radiotherapy plus hyperthermia in locally advanced pelvic tumours: a prospective, randomised, multicentre trial. Dutch Deep Hyperthermia Group. Lancet 2000;355: 1119-1125.

27. Wittlinger M, Rödel CM, Weiss C, et al. Quadrimodal treatment of high-risk T1 and T2 bladder cancer: transurethral tumor resection followed by concurrent radiochemotherapy and regional deep hyperthermia. Radiother Oncol 2009;93:358-63.

28. Merten R, Ott OJ, Haderlein M, et al. Long-term experience of chemoradiotherapy combined with deep regional hyperthermia for organ preservation in high-risk bladder cancer (Ta, Tis, T1, T2). Oncologist 2019;24: e1341-e1350.

29. Goertzen S. Organ-preserving chemoradiation with 5-FU and Cisplatin with and without deep regional hyperthermia for bladder cancer. Erlangen: Friedrich-Alexander University; 2021 Available at: https:// opus4.kobv.de/opus4-fau/frontdoor/index/index/docId/ 15780

30. Riesterer O, Ademaj A, Puric E, et al. Tetramodal therapy with transurethral resection followed by chemoradiation in combination with hyperthermia for muscle-invasive bladder cancer: early results of a multicenter phase IIB study. Int J Hyperthermia 2022;39:1078-1087.

31. Hu Y, Li Z, Mi D-H, et al. Chemoradiation combined with regional hyperthermia for advanced oesophageal cancer: a systematic review and meta-analysis. J Clin Pharm Ther2017;42:155-164.

4. The Role of Hyperthermia in Pediatric Oncology

4.1. Indications

Today, it is estimated that more than 80% of children and adolescents diagnosed with cancer can be successfully treated with established standard therapy according to pediatric oncology protocols [1-2]. Prior to the 2000s, the improvement in survival was primarily due to intensification of therapy, particularly for high-risk patient populations, and advances in supportive care. However, in recent years, the improvement in survival rates for children with cancer has slowed. Therefore, with increasing availability, targeted small molecule and immunotherapeutic agents – beside some hyperthermia programs – will play an increasing role in pediatric cancer clinical trials in the future, but are currently still in the clinical development [3]. Because of the actual cure rates and the present limitations of radiofrequency hyperthermia to single body regions (at this time tumors in areas of the brain and the lungs cannot be treated in children and adolescents), a careful review of the indication is necessary (☞ Figure 4.1). At present, only a limited number of children and adolescents per year are considered for regional hyperthermia, due to the low number of children and adolescents with malignant tumors and the early development of distant metastases [4].

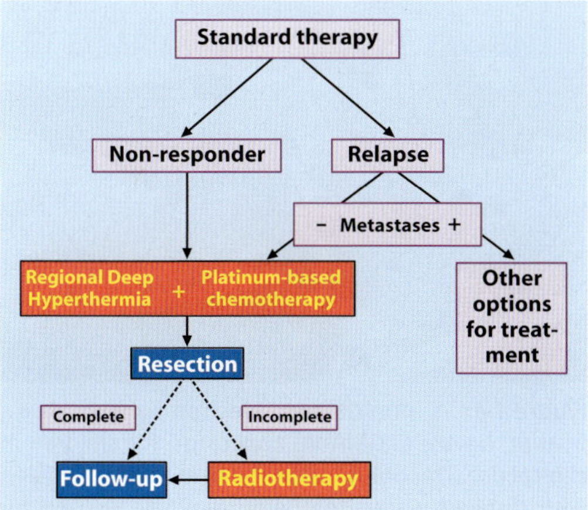

Figure 4.1: An algorithm for regional deep hyperthermia in children and adolescents with malignant tumors. When single metastases can be eradicated by surgery and/or radiotherapy, patients can also be evaluated for regional hyperthermia treatment.

Locoregional hyperthermia is used in children and adolescents to facilitate, rather than replace, surgical tumor resection and/or radiotherapy. Therefore, special multidisciplinary consultations are necessary before the implementation of heat treatment. The usage of locoregional hyperthermia in childhood cancers is always planned under curative aims. Therefore, appropriate staging examinations have to be conducted prior to treatment. The need for repeated treatment courses also makes the general clinical condition, Karnofsky score ≥70% and sufficient hematopoietic regeneration after chemotherapy, other important prerequisites for treatment indication. Regarding the present standard of knowledge, a substantial diminution of the chemotherapy dosage (>20-30%) leads to a clear reduction in the likelihood of treatment success [5-7]. Therefore, the collection of peripheral stem cells is mandatory after intensive courses of chemotherapy. The Hyper-PEI protocol for the application of locoregional hyperthermia at tumor temperatures of 42-44°C in combination with systemic chemotherapy is designed for children and adolescents who suffer from a non-responding, unresectable, or recurrent tumor without distant metastases (for details, ☞ Section 4.2.3). Predominantly germ cell tumors and rhabdomyosarcomas are considered in this protocol, particularly in patients with refractory or recurrent tumors. In addition to these indications for the Hyper-PEI protocol, other methods such as hyperthermic intraperitoneal chemoperfusion (HIPEC) and isolated limb perfusion (ILP) are increasingly used in unfavorable located RMS and other soft tissue tumors like DSRCT in the abdomen or extremities.

4.2. Locoregional Radiofrequency Hyperthermia in Children and Adolescents

4.2.1. Application of Hyperthermia and Thermometry

To apply regional deep hyperthermia (RHT) to children and adolescents with different body dimensions, three electromagnetic heat applicators constructed in the same way are used (☞ Figure 4.2). All standard applicators (Pyrexar Medical

Inc, Salt Lake City, Utah, USA) are comprised of eight bipolar antennae, which are arranged equidistantly in a circle, inside a lucite cylinder with a diameter of 28 cm, 40 cm or 60 cm. With a power supply of 10 to 20 W/kg body weight and frequencies of 90 to 170 MHz, electromagnetic wave heating produces temperatures between 42°C and 44°C. Temperatures are measured in all children and adolescents with nonpertubing thermometers (Bowman probes) at fixed points, including the bladder (abdominal and pelvic tumors) and various critical skin areas [7]. In addition, temperature distribution is measured in the tumor area and the surrounding normal tissue, as well as in the vagina and rectum in cases of abdominal and pelvic tumors, by multipoint thermometry approximately every 5 minutes using an automatic mapping system (Pyrexar Medical Inc, Salt Lake City, Utah). Patients with head and neck tumors are treated with the SA-115 applicator (single spiral antenna, 180-190 MHz) or the SA-mini-spiral applicator. In these cases, temperature measurement is performed with tumor and skin probes only. Calibration of all thermometers is within 0.1°C of the National Bureau of Standards traceable standard thermistors. Details of local radiofrequency hyperthermia technique and temperature monitoring in children are described in Figures 4.3 and 4.4.

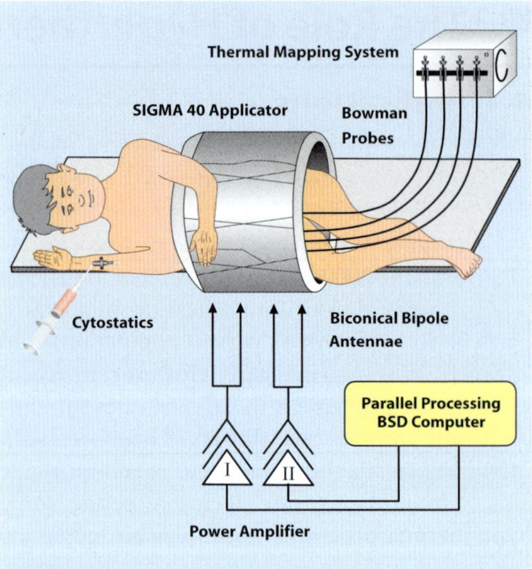

Figure 4.3: Two power amplifiers are shown steering eight bipolar antennae inside a lucite cylinder. Electromagnetic waves are focused on the tumor area. Intratumoral and surrounding normal tissue temperature is measured with nonperturbing Bowman probes. When the intratumoral temperature reaches 42°C, cytostatic drugs are applied as short term infusions according to the hyper-PEI protocol.

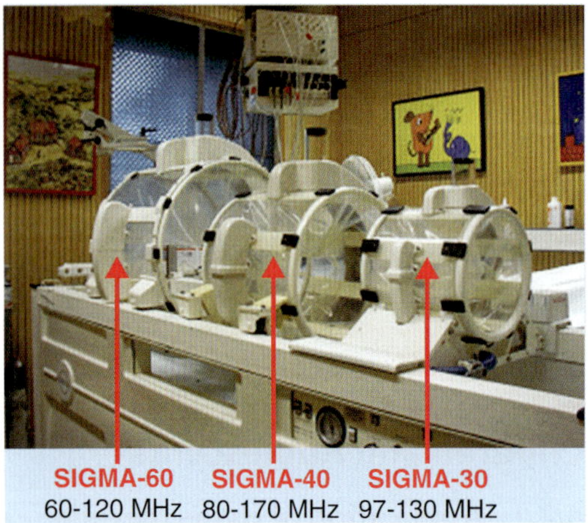

Figure 4.2: The generation of locoregional hyperthermia in infants and children requires different heat applicator equipment from that used in adolescents and adults.

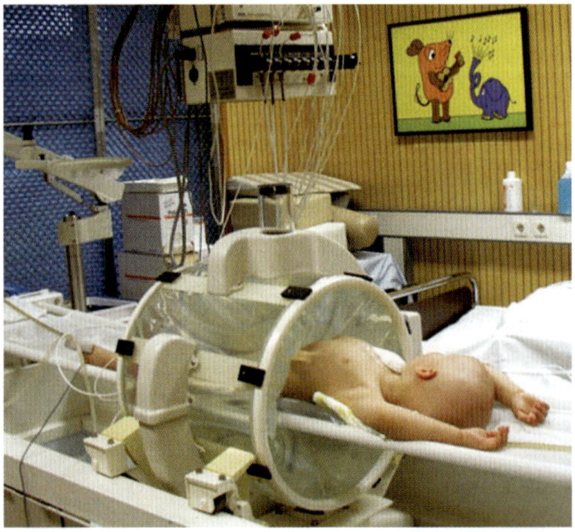

Figure 4.4: A noninvasive electromagnetic deep-heating device (SIGMA-40 applicator) for children in clinical use. The bolus inside the heat applicator filled with distilled water (temperature, 25°C) is used for electromagnetic coupling and body surface cooling. To avoid hot spot phenomena on the patient's back (dorsal position in the applicator) the patient is placed on water cushions connected to a cooling system (thermostat temperature = 20°C).

4.2.2. Analysis of Temperatures

Extensive temperature monitoring is mandatory in order to perform regional deep hyperthermia in children and adolescents with sedation [6, 7]. End-closed plastic catheters are implanted, either by CT guidance or by minimally invasive surgical intervention, to record temperatures in the tumor as well as in neighboring normal tissues. For thermal analysis, temperature files of the parallel processing computer are transferred to an MS-ACCESS database that could be viewed by the ODBC (Open Data Base Connectivity) as statistical analysis system files (SPSS Statistics, release 29.0, IBM, Chicago, IL). In the SPSS program, all temperature records during the treatment time (excluding the warming-up period) in the tumor area and the surrounding normal tissue are calculated as the mean ± standard deviation of T_{min}, T_{90} (10th percentile), T_{50} (50th percentile), T_{20} (80th percentile), and T_{max} per patient. The thermal isoeffect dose method of the Arrhenius relation is also used to convert the time-temperature results in the tumor area to an equivalent number of minutes at a standard temperature (43°C), in which

$$CEM_{43^\circ C}T_{90} = \sum(\Delta t)R(43^\circ C - T),$$

with $CEM_{43^\circ C}T_{90}$ equal to cumulative equivalent minutes at a T_{90} converted to 43°C, Δt equal to the time increments at which data are acquired during treatment, T equal to the average temperature over the time interval Δt, and R equal to 0.25 when $T<43°C$ and 0.5 when $T=43°C$ [8-11]. In the meantime, extensive comparative investigations show that radiofrequency hyperthermia can also be applied with sufficient safety to infants and children, leading to intratumoral temperatures that can be correlated with the same temperatures that are predictive of an improvement of survival in adults (☞ Figure 4.5). Apart from the attainable maximum temperatures of 42-44°C, the measured temperatures of 41.3°C for T_{50} and of 39.4 and/or 40.4°C for T_{90}, as well as $CEM_{43^\circ C}T_{90}$ >5 minutes in the children under 5 years of age and between 5 and 15 years of age are of importance, since the lowest intratumoral temperatures are also essential for prognosis [7].

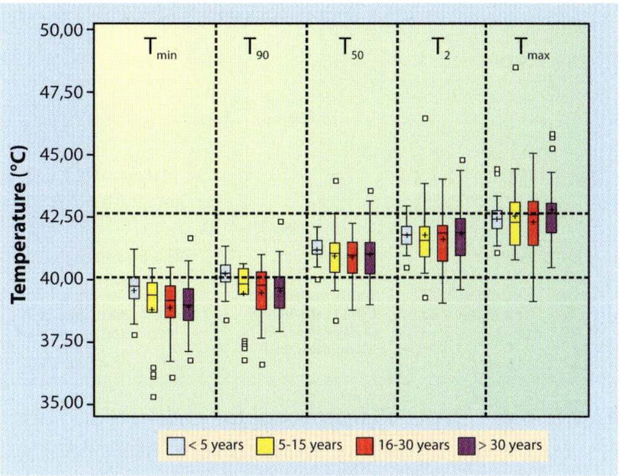

Figure 4.5: Temperature distribution in the tumor and neighboring normal tissue with respect to the position of the thermistor catheter in the tissue at the area of application of regional deep hyperthermia. To assess treatment quality, the temperature measurements of T_{max}, T_{50}, T_{90} and T_{min} in the tumor area and the neighboring normal tissue must be determined.

4.2.3. Hyper-PEI Treatment Schedule

Children and adolescents are sedated before each RHT treatment with midazolam (0.25 mg/kg intravenous [IV]), promethazine hydrochloride (0.05 mg/kg IV), dehydrobenzperidole (0.5 mg/kg IV), and pethidine (0.5 mg/kg IV). Supplemental doses of these drugs are given every 15-30 minutes to maintain sedation [6, 12]. Due to these preventive measures, the presence of an intensive-care experienced pediatrician who continually supervises vital parameters, including transcutaneous oxygen saturation, is always necessary. Multidrug chemotherapy is comprised of cisplatin (40 mg/m^2 IV) on days 1 and 4, etoposide (100 mg/m^2 IV) on days 1-4, and ifosfamide (1800 mg/m^2 IV) on days 1-4. In resistant soft tissue sarcomas cisplatin is replaced by doxorubicin (30 mg/m^2 IV) on days 1 and 4 (☞ Figure 4.6).

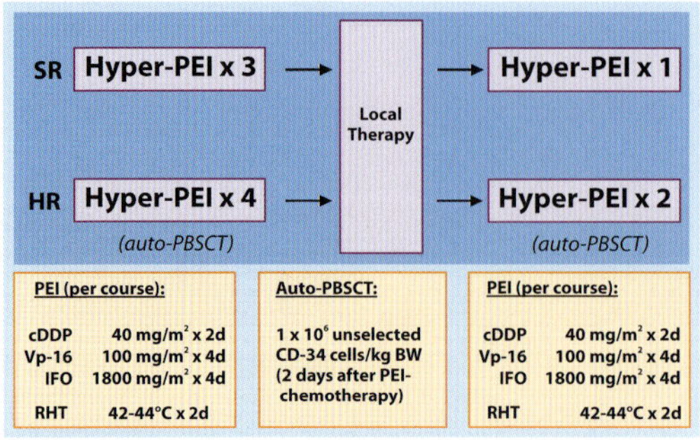

Figure 4.6: Hyper-PEI-protocol for children and adolescents with refractory or recurrent malignancies: Two different risk groups are defined. Patients with refractory or recurrent germ cell tumors are treated with 4 Hyper-PEI courses in the standard risk arm (SR). Patients with poor prognostic tumors, including refractory sarcomas, are treated in the high-risk arm (HR) with 6 Hyper-PEI courses. In platinum-resistant cases replacement by doxorubicin is scheduled. After intensive chemotherapy pre-treatment stem cells must be harvested for these treatment schedules.

After a warming-up period of 30 minutes, cytostatic drugs are administered on days 1 and 4 as short-term infusions into a Broviac catheter simultaneously with 1 hour of RHT. Bladder cooling during hyperthermia is performed with distilled water as soon as the intravesical temperature exceeds 42.5°C. To avoid vesical hemorrhage, mesnauro protection is used for 5 days, beginning at the same time as ifosfamide application. To reduce cisplatin-based nephrotoxicity, mannitol diuresis is performed 6, 3, and 0.5 hours before and after cisplatin application. All patients receive antiemetics comprised of ondansetron (8 mg/m^2 daily) for 5 days, by 24-hour infusion. Chemotherapy cycles are scheduled at 21-day intervals. Cisplatin is reduced by 50% if the glomerular filtration rate is <60 mL/minute or replaced by equivalent doses of carboplatin. Chemotherapy is delayed for 1 or 2 weeks in patients with a leukocyte count <2000/mL, a platelet count <80,000/mL, or a Karnofsky performance status <70%. During the entire treatment period, the patients receive prophylactic antibiotics against pneumocystis with trimethomoprim/sulfamethoxazole (3 × 5/20 mg/kg per week) [6, 13].

4.3. Limitations

The predominant patient risks arise from the highly dosed chemotherapeutics, which correspond to those of other pediatric study protocols. Moreover, it must be taken into account that cisplatin-induced nephrotoxicity is increased when treatments of the central and upper abdomen are performed [6]. In this situation a dose reduction of cisplatin or its replacement by carboplatin may be required in the treatment schedule. In principle, using additional heat treatment for local tumor control puts the skin and deeper tissues at risk of thermal damage. In addition, hip necrosis is occasionally found in the multimodal approach of the Hyper-PEI-protocol (☞ Figure 4.7), and can also be caused by the hyperthermia treatment [6, 13]. Optimizing treatment applications, continuous invasive temperature monitoring, and the use of optimized annular phased array systems in infants and children with sedation can minimize thermal tissue damage (degree II, III <1%) [8]. In this context, contraindications for the application of radiofrequency hyperthermia must be taken into account. Such contraindications include metal implants, which can cause extreme high temperatures, and electronic components, which can be perturbed.

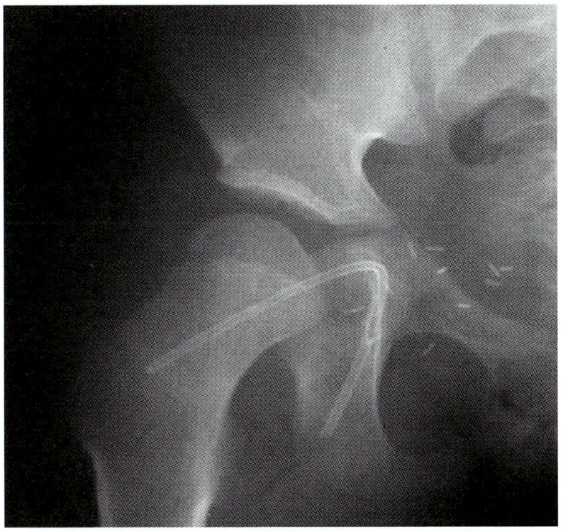

a

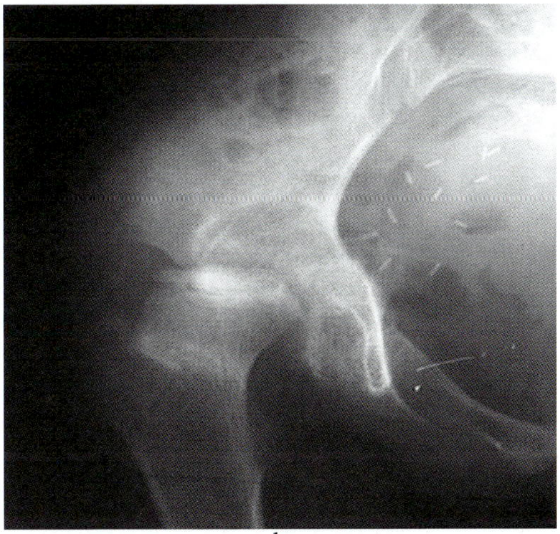

b

Figure 4.7: X-ray of the normal right hip in a 4-year-old boy before beginning hyperthermia treatment (**a**). Seven months after thermochemotherapy, an aseptic osteonecrosis (AON) of the right hip was found (**b**).

4.4. Results

4.4.1. Experimental Studies

Before routine clinical use of hyperthermia in standardized protocols, numerous experimental laboratory examinations demonstrated that the cytostatic effects of anticancer drugs can be significantly increased by additional hyperthermia at temperatures between 40°C and 44°C [14-16]. These thermal effects have also been shown with respect to cell lines of childhood cancers, including germ cell tumors, neuroblastomas, osteosarcomas, and Ewing's sarcomas [17-18]. For example, various human Ewing's sarcoma cell lines have revealed a very different sensibility against cisplatin at a temperature of 37°C. However, a marked increase in the anti-cancer effects of cisplatin can be demonstrated at temperatures ranging from 41°C to 43°C (☞ Figure 4.8). In regards to these results, it must be recognized that anti-cancer drugs that are effective under hyperthermic conditions do not necessarily have the same level of effectiveness in standard therapy performed at normal body temperature. A further example for the overcoming of resistance mechanisms by hyperthermia is given by the cisplatin-resistant JAR choriocarcinoma cell line, on which cisplatin has a dose-dependent anticancer effect at elevated temperatures of 42°C and 43°C (☞ Figure 4.9).

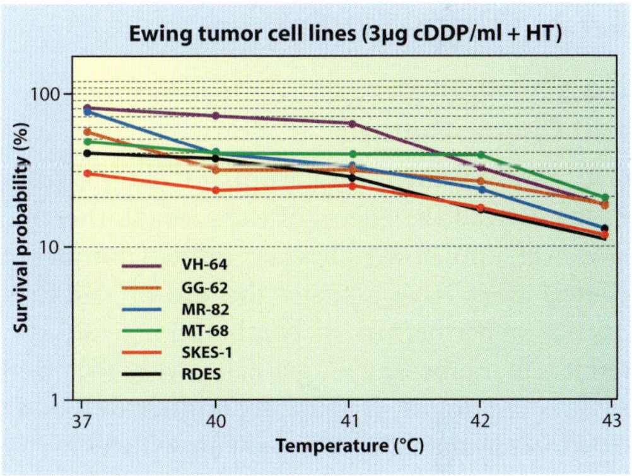

Figure 4.8: Effects of chemotherapy with cisplatin (cDDP) and heat treatment (HT) on six human Ewing sarcoma cell lines: HT at temperatures between 41.0°C and 43.0°C increases the effects of cDDP at a dosage of 3 µg/mL.

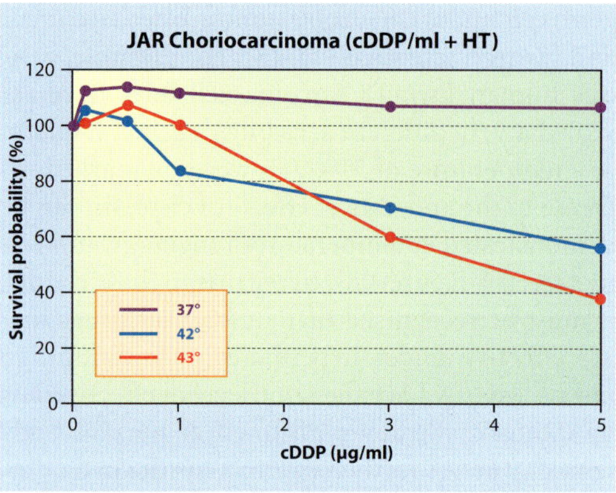

Figure 4.9: JAR choriocarcinoma cell line: At a temperature of 37°C (blue line) the JAR cell line is resistant to chemotherapy with cisplatin (cDDP). The JAR cell line is diminished by the same cDDP dosage at temperatures of 42°C (green line) or 43°C (red line), demonstrating that cDDP-resistance can overcome by heat.

4.4.2. Clinical Studies

4.4.2.1. Radiofrequency Hyperthermia and Chemotherapy

Over the past three decades, many clinical trials have analyzed the effects of thermoradiotherapy. However, until now, only a very limited number of clinical trials have assessed the use of radiofrequency hyperthermia in combination with systemic chemotherapy in patients with localized tumors. Therefore, a phase III multicenter study (RHT 96) by the EORTC in patients with high-risk soft tissue sarcomas is notable, particularly because it analyzes the effectiveness of additional neoadjuvant locoregional deep hyperthermia in comparison to conventional treatment options such as chemotherapy, surgery, and/or radiotherapy [19-20]. In this phase III study, the application of additional hyperthermia in this high-risk sarcoma patient population was found to have prognostic value for better local tumor control and longer event-free and overall survival [21-22].

Due to encouraging results in adults with recurrent or advanced tumors, children and adolescents were also treated with these treatment modalities, after all established therapeutic options had been exhausted without success. First, generated treatment data were collected and evaluated under uniform criteria by Romanowski et al. In this early phase of additional heat application, a tumor response was found in six out of 34 intensively pretreated patients <18 years of age. These preliminary results demonstrated the fundamental applicability of the method [23].

In a consecutive phase-II study at the Heinrich Heine University, we treated refractory childhood cancers with diverse histopathological patterns according to standardized systemic PEI-chemotherapy and regional deep hyperthermia (42-44°C) in order to examine tumor response and options of complete tumor resection. A total of 39 patients have been enrolled onto this phase II study (12 months 37.5 years, median 5.2 years). Among these, 24 patients had extracranial non-testicular germ cell tumors and 15 patients soft tissue or chondrosarcomas. Indication was locoregional relapse (n=29) or unresectable tumor after neoadjuvant chemotherapy (n=10). Among these two groups, there were ten patients with poor response or progressive disease under primary or relapse chemotherapy. Ten out of the 29 relapse patients had more than one relapse. Twenty patients achieved complete response after thermochemotherapy (TCH), and ten patients achieved partial response. TCH was followed by surgical tumor resection in 28/39 patients and/or radiotherapy in 13/39 patients. At a median follow-up of 27 months, five-year event-free (EFS) and overall survival (OS) for the whole study cohort was 0.39 ± 0.11 (20/39 patients) and 0.52 ± 0.11 (25/39 patients), respectively. TCH shows substantial therapeutic efficacy and facilitates complete tumor resection in 14 out of 28 operated patients. This multimodal treatment regimen including TCH, surgical resection and/or radiotherapy leads to sustained remission in the majority of patients with refractory locoregional tumors. These data formed the basis for the current pediatric hyperthermia study and were integrated into a prospective treatment optimization trial (Hyper-PEI) for the treatment of children with refractory or recurrent solid tumors. The central inclusion criterion for the

Hyper-PEI protocol is the presence of a malignant solid extracranial tumor that is refractory to conventional treatment or presents as an unresectable locoregional relapse. Patients with metastases may also be included, if the anatomic situation suggests that the treatment of the tumor area will achieve a therapeutic effect on both the tumor and the metastases [13].

Within the scope of this ongoing Hyper-PEI protocol, which is registered at the German Cancer Society, a cohort of 44 patients (7 months to 21 years; median 2.7 years) with refractory or recurrent malignant germ-cell tumors was prospectively analyzed. The primary endpoint was the proportion of patients who had an objective response as assessed with Response Evaluation Criteria in Solid Tumors (RECIST 1.0 guidelines). Secondary endpoints were the event-free survival and overall survival after 5 years. We identified 34 yolk sac tumors, eight embryonal carcinomas, one choriocarcinoma, and one dysgerminoma by histology analysis. Of the 35 patients who had sufficient clinical and radiographical data available for response assessment, 30 (86%) had an objective response to treatment (16 patients had CR and 14 had PR). 5-year event-free survival was 62%, and 5-year overall survival was 72%. Subgroup analysis showed apparently better survival in patients who received PEI-chemotherapy and regional deep hyperthermia as a salvage therapy for a poor response or a first relapse than in patients with multiple relapses (☞ Figure 4.12).

Acute toxic effects were assessed in all 44 patients with 181 Hyper-PEI cycles. Myelotoxic effects were similar to those noted in other intensive chemotherapy regimens used to treat childhood cancer. Grade 3-4 neutropenia occurred in all chemotherapy cycles. Granulocytopenic fever, which required intercurrent hospital admission, was noted in 29 (66%) of 44patients after 53 (29%) of 181 chemotherapy cycles; these patients were treated with intravenous antibiotics. We recorded thrombocytopenia of grade 3-4 after all cycles. No major bleeding occurred, and we noted no peripheral neuropathy. Nausea and emesis were generally mild to moderate and more pronounced in older patients than in infants and toddlers. Nine patients received cyclophosphamide (360 mg/m² per day on days 1-4) instead of ifosfamide; two of these patients were younger than 2 years of age, and four had symptoms of ifosfamide-induced encephalopathy, either before (two patients) or during (two patients) PEI-regional deep hyperthermia. Three of these patients had grade 3 renal tubular damage. Grade 1 mild skin inflammation occurred in the treatment area of five patients after 21 heat sessions but resolved fully within 3 days. Grade 2 anogenital blisters occurred in two patients after two sessions but healed within 1-2 weeks; no severe skin bums were noted. Mild-to-moderate grade 1 pain, described as muscle aching, was reported in the bones and muscles of the treated area of seven patients after 22 sessions. Two patients had aseptic necrosis of the left femoral head, which required orthopedic intervention at 2 or 4 months after the end of regional deep hyperthermia treatment [24].

For another larger series (n=23) of our Hyper-PEI patient population with refractory and recurrent rhabdomyosarcomas (RMS), Kaplan Maier survival curve (overall survival, OS) is documented. Survival was encouraging among patients suffering from unresectable sarcomas, with an OS rate of 0.67±0.19, while only 3 of 11 patients with RMS relapses survived (☞ Figure 4.13).

4.4.2.2. Radiofrequency Hyperthermia and Radiotherapy

To date, no controlled trial results exist on the use of RHT with radiotherapy (thermoradiotherapy) in pediatric tumor patients, although adult studies have shown improvement in local tumor control and overall survival with additional RHT. The Dutch Deep Hyperthermia Trial not only showed an 83% local control rate for combined radiation therapy and RHT versus 57% for radiation therapy alone, but also a 3-year OS of 51% for radiation therapy combined with RHT, compared to 27% with radiation therapy alone. The 12-year OS was still almost twice as high after combined radiation therapy and RHT (37%), versus 20% with radiation therapy alone [25]. Nevertheless, limited experience in individual cases provides evidence in pediatric tumor patients that thermoradiotherapy may have the same synergistic effects as in adults. Overall, we now survey the treatments of 19 children and adolescents aged between 0.7 and 17.9 years (median: 3.11 years) with refractory or recurrent malignant tumors (five patients with poor response, 4 patients with first relapse, 10 patients with multiple relapses). We identified 10 malignant germ cell tumors, 8 rhabdomyosarcomas and one nephroblastoma by histology analysis. All patients received external radiotherapy of 19,2-51,6 Gy (median total dose 49.6 Gy), 1.6-2.4 Gy per fraction (five times per week) in combination with 1-hour regional hyperthermia at 42-44°C (day 1+5 per week). The time difference between irradiation and the onset of hyperthermia was 30 minutes (mean). There was only grade 1-2 acute toxicity at the skin detected. One of 6 long-term survivors suffered from an avascular osteonecrosis of the femoral head which required surgical intervention. These preliminary data merits further investigation to evaluate the outcome and toxicities of thermoradiotherapy in pediatric patients.

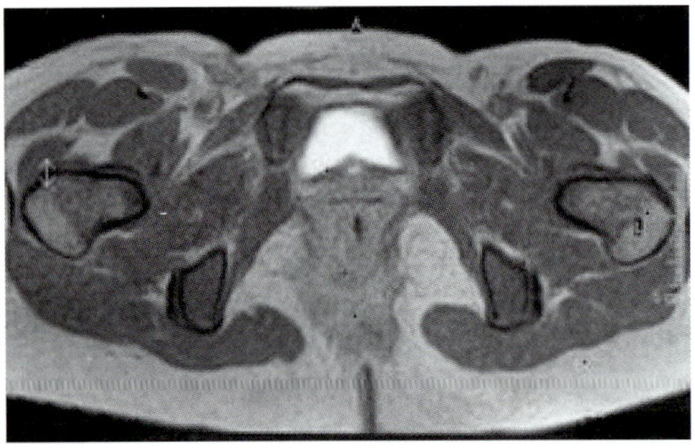

a

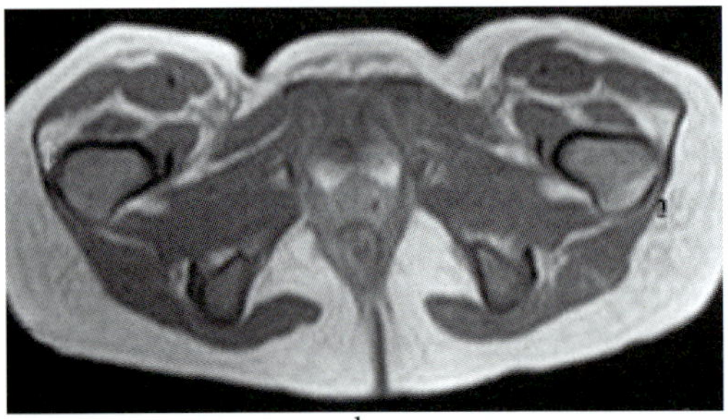

b

Figure 4.10: Magnetic resonance imaging (MRI) of the pelvis showing an embryonal rhabdomyosarcoma (RMS) in the anal region (18-year-old patient). The embryonal RMS did not respond to standard chemotherapy (**a**). Complete regression of the embryonal RMS was achieved after three courses of PEI-chemotherapy in combination with regional deep hyperthermia according to the Hyper-PEI protocol (**b**).

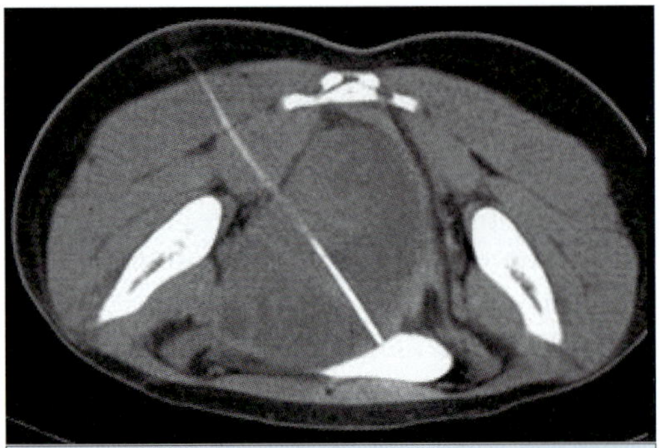

Start RHT	
	Median
$CEM_{43°C}T_{90}$	73.4
T_{90}	41.5
T_{50}	43.6
T_{max}	45.0

a

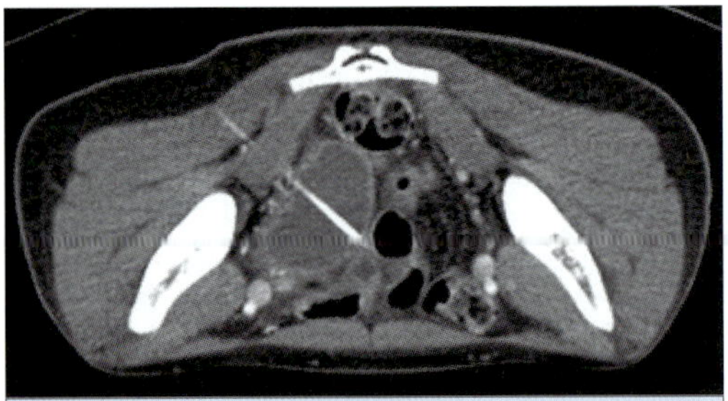

10 weeks later

Hyper-PEI × 4

b

Figure 4.11: 13-year-old female patient. Computed tomography (CT) reveals a non-resectable Sertoli-Leydig-cell tumor (**a**) in the pelvis. The tumor did not respond to standard chemotherapy. Marked tumor regression was observed after four courses of PEI chemotherapy in combination with regional deep hyperthermia according to the Hyper-PEI protocol (**b**). Invasive temperature monitoring revealed tumor temperatures for T^{90} and T_{max} between 41.5°C and 45.0°C.

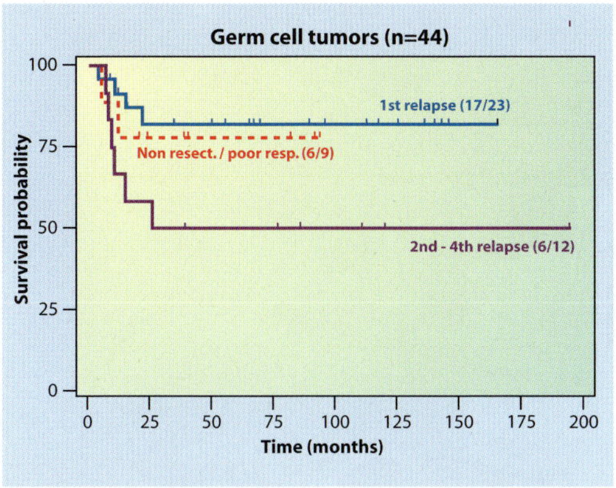

Figure 4.12: Kaplan-Maier analysis in children and adolescents with refractory germ cell tumors (GCT) after standard therapy. After treatment according to the hyper-PEI protocol, the survival probability for patients with non-resectable, non-responding, or first GCT relapse is significantly better than for patients with 2-4 GCT relapses.

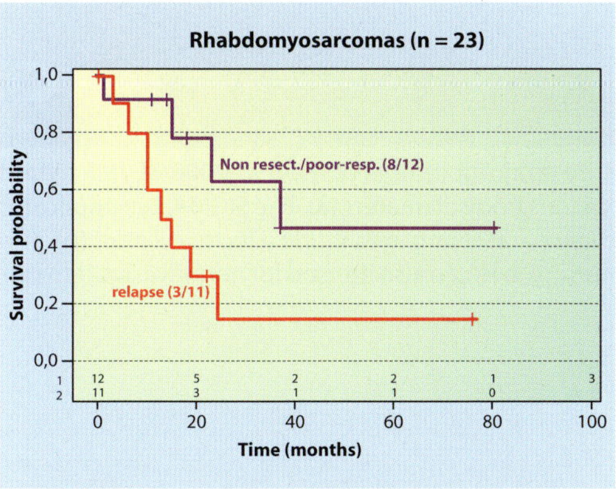

Figure 4.13: Kaplan-Maier analysis in children and adolescents with refractory rhabdomyosarcomas (RMS) after standard therapy. After treatment according to the hyper-PEI protocol the survival probabilitiy for patients with non-resectable or non-responding RMS tumors is significantly better than for patients with RMS relapses.

By employing multimodal concepts with regional hyperthermia, the objective of local tumor control and durable remission can be obtained in children with high-risk tumors with unfavorable prognosis. In the future, additional use of 3D multiple channel heat applicators and non-invasive MR temperature monitoring for childhood cancers gives hope for a precise imaging of the affected tissue as well as neighboring healthy tissue – even in infants and children.

4.5. Technical Approach and Perspectives

The realization that only optimum technology could obtain therapeutic successes with tolerable side effects led to a progressive development of the required technologies, and to the optimization of heat application and temperature measurement in children and adolescents. In order to sufficiently treat children and adolescents with different tumor sizes or disseminated abdominal tumors, various electromagnetic applicators with 8-24 bipolar antennae in two- or three-dimensional arrangement for locoregional hyperthermia are currently being tested. These innovations are expected to result in a higher and more homogeneous temperature distribution in the tumor area [26]. This generation of radiofrequency applicators (BSD-2000/3D/MR hybrid system) can be integrated into 1.5-Tesla MRT systems, making simultaneous non-invasive temperature measurements possible (☞ Figure 4.14). In the future, it is important that new software programs are available, to optimise hyperthermia treatment settings of radiofrequency antennas by computer simulation (treatment planning) and to correct artifactual MR images for exact temperature recording [27-28]. An example of non-invasive temperature monitoring by MRI in comparison to invasive thermometry by Bowman probes is given in Figure 4.15 and Figure 4.16. The integration of phase and amplitude evaluation at the feed points, advanced phantoms, and precise positioning into current and future QA procedures should be evaluated to guarantee the best possible quality of patient care [29].

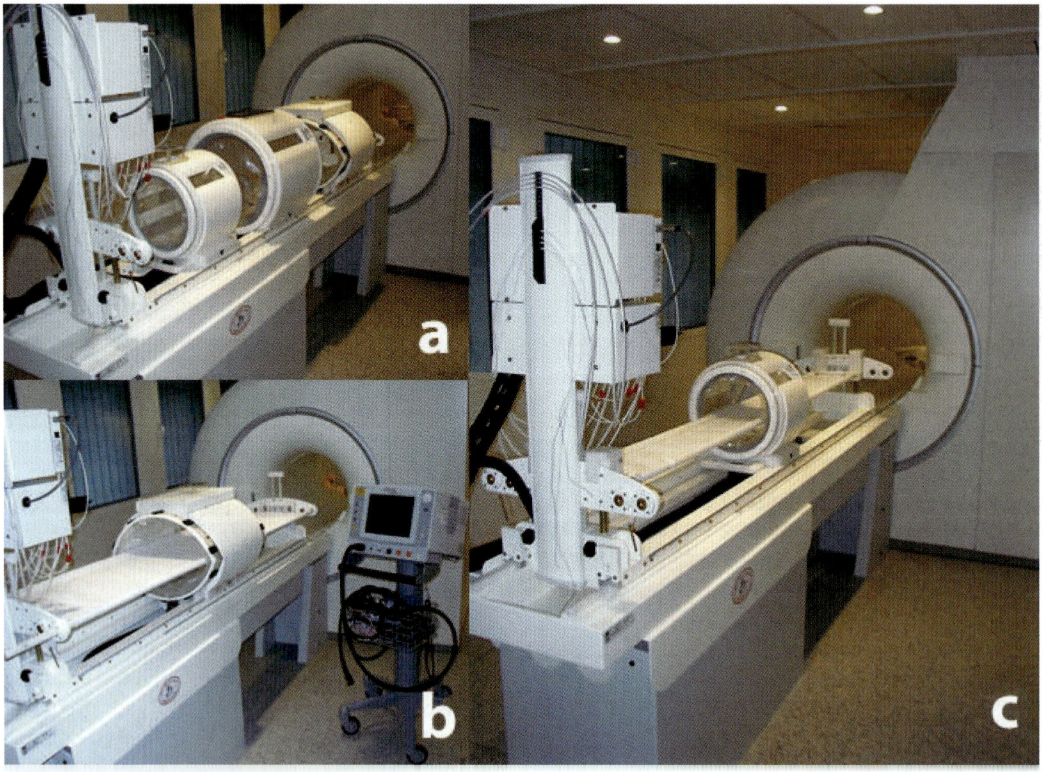

Figure 4.14: Three different electromagnetic annular phased array applicators of the BSD-2000/3D/MR hybrid system for the treatment of children and adolescents with various body diameters (**a**). The SIGMA-Eye applicator consists of 24 bipolar antennae arranged equidistantly in three parallel ring axes inside a lucite cylinder (**b**). The SIGMA-30 MR, which consists of eight bipolar antennae in one ring axis, can also be used for non-invasive temperature monitoring inside the 1.5-Tesla Symphony MRI (**c**).

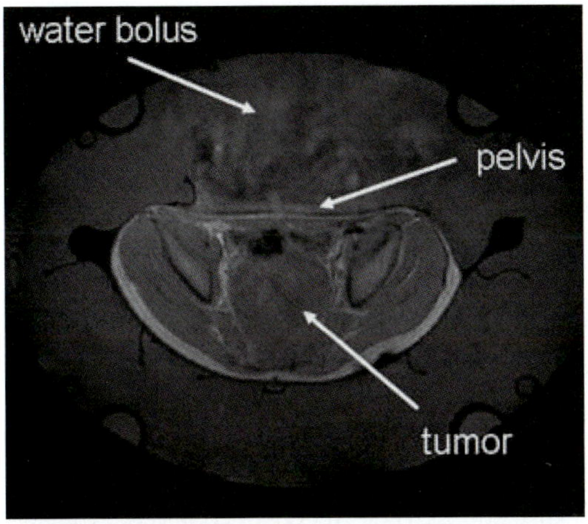

a

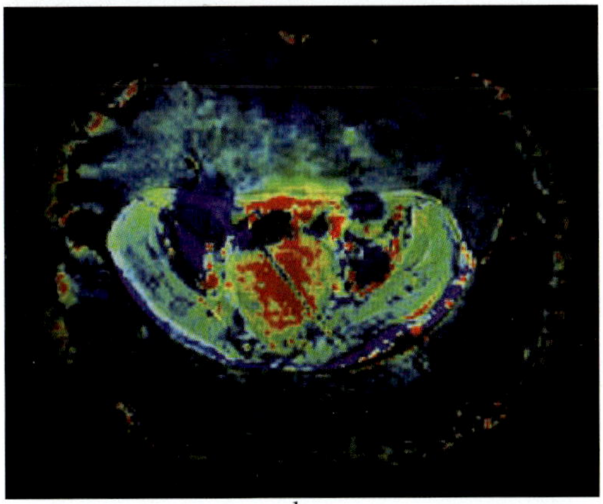

b

Figure 4.15: Magnetic resonance imaging (MRI) shows a large pelvic germ cell tumor and the water bolus of the SIGMA-Eye heat applicator (**a**). The SigmaVision computer program (Dr. Sennewald Medizintechnik GmbH, Munich, Germany) of the BSD-2000/3D/MR hybrid system can transform T1-relaxation signals in temperature-dependent colors to allow monitoring of tissue temperature (**b**).

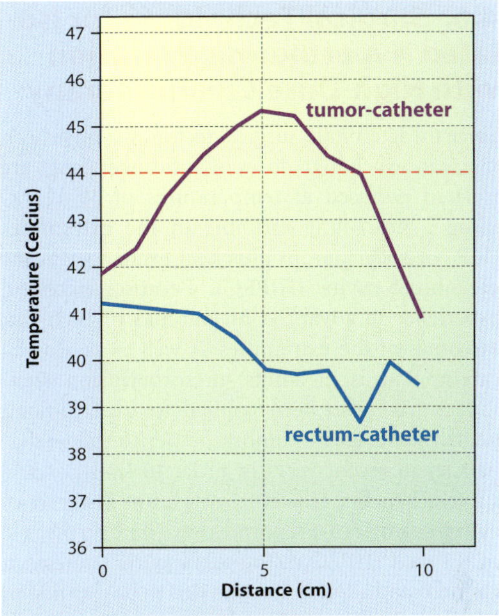

a

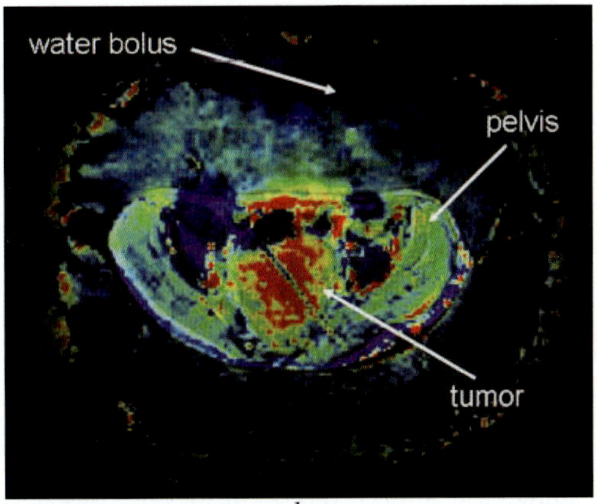

b

Figure 4.16: Correlation of invasive thermometry by nonperturbing Bowman probes (**a**) with noninvasive MR signals (**b**) in the pelvis area.

4.6. Surgical Techniques for Isolated Hyperthermic Perfusion with High-Dose Chemotherapy

Since the late 1960s, surgical techniques have been in use in which high doses of anticancer drugs are isolated perfused at temperatures of 39-42.5°C using a heart-lung machine in the extremities (ILP) or roller pumps plus heat exchanger in the abdominal cavity (HIPEC). Because successful experience in advanced melanomas or high-risk sarcomas of the extremities as well as peritoneal carcinomatosis in adults, these perfusion techniques have also been applied to treat difficult pediatric extremity tumors or peritoneal malignancies in recent years in order to find possible survival benefits. However, only limited case series as well as single case reports exist to date, so the role of ILP and HIPEC in the therapeutic strategy in children and adolescents remains to be clarified in future trials. Nevertheless, it is important to know the most widely accepted indications so that uniform strategies can be followed in the future and registered in appropriate databases.

4.6.1. Isolated Hyperthermic Limb Perfusion

After Creech and Krementz introduced isolated limb perfusion with melphalan (L-PAM) for the treatment of metastatic malignant melanomas and locally advanced high-risk sarcomas in adults, the addition of heat at temperatures between 39-42°C and recombinant tumor necrosis factor α (TNFα) have revolutionized tumor response and long-term outcome [30-33]. Reasonable at the histopathological level TNFα induces microvascular damage through loss of endothelial cohesion and therefore the addition of TNFα to the perfusate results in a significant increase in drug uptake of L-PAM or doxorubicin by tumors [34]. The fact that limb-preserving surgery after hyperthermic ILP over 60-90 minutes with L-PAM ± TNFα is equal to amputation in terms of overall survival, stimulated the use of this concept in selected children and adolescents with extended limb tumors.

In an early process phase six children (12-16 years) and eight adolescents (16-20 years) with extremity melanomas were included in an ILP program before wide tumor excision was performed [35]. The median Breslow thickness of the melanomas was 2.7 mm (range, 1 to 15 mm). Hyperthermic isolated limb perfusion was performed with L-PAM (10 mg/L extremity volume) over 60 minutes perfusion time at a temperature of 39-40°C. The median follow-up period was approximately 10 years. Distant metastases developed in three patients (one patient was in Stage IA) and two patients were in Stage IIIB). In two cases the development of distant metastases was preceded by local recurrence. The 5-year survival rate was 93%. The high survival rate, even for patients with unfavorably thick melanomas, seems to be attributable to isolated regional perfusion.

Hohenberger and Tunn performed ILP with 2 mg TNFα followed by L-PAM (10 mg/L extremity volume) over 90 minutes perfusion time with a maximum tumor temperature of 39.2°C in two children with synovial sarcoma recurrences.

- 1) An 8-year-old boy with a biphasic, fibroblastic synovial sarcoma of intermediate grade. Local recurrence occurred after adjuvant VAIA chemotherapy (vincristine, adriamycin, ifosfamide, and actinomycin D), resection and 45 Gy of adjuvant radiotherapy.
- 2) A 11 year old girl suffered from a locally recurrent synovial sarcoma at the anterior distal part of her left ankle. She also received adjuvant VAIA chemotherapy, tumor resection and radiotherapy of 44.6 Gy to the area of the primary tumor.

As consequence of this ILP therapy all resection specimen revealed extensive necrosis of the tumor in both cases. Morbidity after ILP showed no major disadvantages except subcutaneous fibrosis and mild lymphedema. Although the boy developed twenty-six months after ILP treatment multiple lung metastases, both patients had persistent local tumor control with excellent functional outcomes [36].

4.6.2. Hyperthermic Intraperitoneal Chemoperfusion

Peritoneal malignant tumors are rare in children and have a poor prognosis. Because these high-risk malignancies most often present metastasized in extensive areas of the peritoneum (sarcomatosis), aggressive treatment options are necessary. An effective treatment must eradicate free tumor cells and microscopic disease in the peritoneal cavity after cytoreductive surgery (CRS) to prevent further peritoneal dissemination. In recent years, CRS and HIPEC, as successful local control approaches in adults, have been applied to pediatric peritoneal malignancies.

Desmoplastic small round cell tumors (DSRCT) and rhabdomyosarcomas are the most common pediatric indications today. The pioneering work of Hayes Jordan at the MD Anderson Cancer Center and Fuchs at the University Hospital Tuebingen built the basis for the systematic use of CRS and HIPEC in children. Beside other individual regimens, the abdominal application of 75-100 mg cisplatin/m² (± sodium thiosulfate IV) alone or in combination with 15 mg doxorubicin/m² over a perfusion time of 60-90 minutes (closed abdomen technique) at a temperature of 41-42,5°C is considered suitable, provided that adequate renal and liver function is available. The extent of previous surgical cytoreduction according to the peritoneal carcinomatosis index, as described by Jacquet and Sugarbaker, is decisive for the prognosis. In general, HIPEC should only be offered if complete cytoreduction (CC-0/CC-1; CC-0 meaning no visible disease; CC-1 meaning nodules smaller than 0.25 cm) seems feasible. Consequently, non-resectable liver metastases or extra-abdominal metastases, e.g., in the lungs, represent a contraindication.

The study group of Hayes Jordan was the first, which combined CRS and HIPEC in 8 of 24 patients (5-21 years) with unfavorable abdominal DSRCT. The other patients received systemic chemotherapy alone (n=9) or chemotherapy plus debulking surgery of at least 90% of the tumor (n=7). In comparing those that received CRS with HIPEC versus chemotherapy plus debulking surgery, the 3-year median survivals were 71% and 62%, respectively, and the result was not statistically significant. However, the overall survival in the group who received chemotherapy alone was only 26%, which was statistically significant [37]. The same group conducted a single-arm, single-institution phase II trial in which 20 patients ages 23 months to 50 years, 14 of whom had DSRCT, received CRS and HIPEC. In this highly selected population, the 3-year OS for DSRCT patients was 79%. It should be noted that all DSRCT patients in this study received additional whole abdominal radiation therapy (WART), which may also have contributed to treatment success after CRS and HIPEC [38].

In addition Gesche et al. reported six patients (2-4 years) with initial IRS stage III or IV intra-abdominal embryonal RMS received CRS and HIPEC, with a median follow-up of 12 months (7-41 months). All patients with IRS IV showed complete resolution of extraabdominal metastases at the time of the procedure. HIPEC was performed using cisplatin (37.5-75.0 mg/m²) and doxorubicin (15 mg/m² in the last four patients) for 60 minutes at 42.5 °C. Preoperative staging revealed a primarily disseminated intraperitoneal tumor in two patients. One patient had sustained multifocal tumor recurrence within 6 months after primary treatment and three patients had large intraperitoneal tumor masses upon of diagnosis. Operations comprised extensive peritonectomy procedures and visceral resections including partial cystectomies in two patients, a ureteroureterostomy and a hemicolectomy with primary anastomosis. Complete cytoreduction (CC-0) was achieved in all patients.

In contrast to the considerable side effects described in the literature, no severe (grade 3 or 4 according to the CTCAE) HIPEC-associated toxicities or complications were observed in this cohort. Two patients developed self-limiting proteinuria, which required albumin supplementation and was resolved within days. Mild elevation of renal retention parameters also resolved without reaching critical values for renal insufficiency. In this approach all pediatric patients showed no evidence of disease after 7-41 months follow-up [39]. The significantly lower side effects or complications may be related to the fact that no patient in this study had abdominal radiation prior to HIPEC, as described in previous reports.

4.7. Clinical Aspects

An important task for the future, in cooperation with study leaders in pediatric oncology, is the selection of patient groups with particularly high relapse risk who can profit from additional regional deep hyperthermia, ILP or HIPEC or a combination of these different hyperthermia methods. In these patient groups additional hyperthermia should be implemented as early as possible.

Furthermore, examination of heat-induced biological phenomena is of importance, since it has been shown that tumor infiltrating lymphocytes (TILs), PDL1 and heat shock proteins (HSPs) can cause specific reactions within the immune system and may cause apoptotic cell death or temporary thermal tolerance in tumor cells. In this context, pharmacological targeted therapies, including HSP antibodies or small molecules (e.g., checkpoint inhibitors, quercetin or otherflavonoid compounds), are also of special interest, in addition to the direct interactions of hyperthermia with chemotherapy and/or radiotherapy [40-47].

Acknowledgements

Our hyperthermia projects are supported by grants from the Deutsche Krebshilfe e.V. and the Elterninitivative Kinderkrebsklinik e.V.

4.8. References

1. Adamson PC. Improving the outcome for children with cancer: development of targeted new agents. CA Cancer J Clin 2015;65:212-220.

2. Siegel RL, Miller KD, Wagle NS, Jemal A. Cancer statistics, 2023. CA Cancer J Clin 2023;73(1):17-48.

3. Butler E, Ludwig K, Pacenta HL, Klesse LJ, Watt TC, Laetsch TW. Recent progress in the treatment of cancer in children. CA Cancer J Clin 2021;71(4):315-332.

4. Wessalowski R, Van Heek-Romanowski R, Issels RD, Jürgens H, Göbel U. Estimated number of children eligible for hyperthermia based on population- and treatment-related criteria. Int J Hyperthermia 1999;15:455-466.

5. Van Heek-Romanowski R, D'Oleire F, Havers W. Thermoradiotherapy and thermochemotherapy for pediatric tumors. In M. H. Seegenschmiedt, P. Fessenden, and C. C. Vernon (eds.), Thermoradiotherapy and thermochemotherapy, volume 2: clinical application. Berlin, Heidelberg, New York: Springer Verlag 1995; 187-205.

6. Wessalowski R, Kruck H, Pape H, Kahn T, Willers R, Göbel U. Hyperthermia for the treatment of patients with malignant germ cell tumors: a phase I/II study in ten children and adolescents with recurrent or refractory tumors. Cancer 1998;82:793-800.

7. Wessalowski R. Regionale Tiefenhyperthermie und Chemotherapie bei Tumoren von Kindern und Erwachsenen. Experimentelle und klinische Untersuchungen. Shaker Verlag, Aachen 2002;1-205.

8. Sapareto, S A, Dewey WC. Thermal dose determination in cancer therapy. Int. J Radiat Oncol Biol Phys 1984;10(6):787-800.

9. Oleson JR, Samulski TV, Leopold KA, Clegg ST, Dewhirst MW, Dodge RK, George SL. Sensitivity of hyperthermia trial outcomes to temperature and time: implications for thermal goals of treatment. Int J Radiat Oncol Biol Phys 1993;25(2):289-297.

10. Dewhirst MW. Thermal dosimetry. In MH Seegenschmiedt, P Fessenden, and CC Vernon (eds.), Thermoradiotherapy and Thermochemotherapy, volume 1, biology, physiology, and physics. Berlin, Heidelberg, New York: Springer Verlag 1995;123-136.

11. Dewhirst MW, Oleson JR, Kirkpatrick J, Secomb TW. Accurate three-dimensional thermal dosimetry and assessment of physiologic response are essential for optimizing thermoradiotherapy. Cancers 2022;14(7):1701

12. Wessalowski R, Blohm M, Calaminus G, Engert J, Harms D, Krause I, Kruck H, Grüttner HP, Pape H., Göbel U. Treatment results in children and adolescents with loco-regional recurrences of abdominal germ cell tumors (GCTs): a pilot-study with PEI chemotherapy and regional deep hyperthermia (RHT) in comparison to a matched cohort. Klin Pädiatr 1997; 209(4):250-256.

13. Wessalowski R , Schneider DT, Mils O, Hannen M, Calaminus G, Engelbrecht V, Pape H, Willers R Engert J, Harms D, Göbel U. An approach for cure: PEI-chemotherapy and regional deep hyperthermia in children and adolescents with unresectable malignant tumors. Klin Padiatr 2003; 215(6):303-309.

14. Urano M, Kuroda M, Nishimura Y. For the clinical application of thermochemotherapy given at mild temperatures. Int J Hyperthermia 1999;15(2):79-107.

15. Dahl O. Mechanism of thermal enhancement of chemotherapeutic cytotoxicity. In M Urano and E Douple (eds.), Hyperthermia and oncology, Chemopotention by hyperthermia, volume 4. Utrecht: 1994;9-28.

16. Dahl O. Interaction of heat and drugs in vitro and in vivo. In M. H. Seegenschmiedt, P Fessenden, and CC Vernon (eds.), Thermoradiotherapy and Thermochemotherapy. Berlin, Heidelberg, New York: Springer Verlag 1995;103-121.

17. Debes A, Rommel F, Breise M, Willers R, Göbel U, Wessalowski R. In vitro test-system for chemo- and thermosensitivity: an analysis of survival fractions and cell-cycle distributions in human Ewing's sarcomas as a modelfor tumors in pediatric oncology. Klin Pädiatr 2002;214(4):223-229.

18. Debes A, Willers R, Göbel U, Wessalowski R. Role of heat treatment in childhood cancers: distinct resistance profiles of solid tumor cell lines towards combined thermochemotherapy. Pediatr Blood Cancer 2005;45: 663-669.

19. Issels RD, Prenninger SW, Nagele A, Boehm E, Sauer H, Jauch KW, Denecke H, Berger H, Peter K, Wilmanns

W. Ifosfamide plus etoposide combined with regional hyperthermia in patients with locally advanced sarcomas: a phase II study. J Clin Oncol 1990; 8(11):1818-1829.

20. Issels RD, Abdel-Rahman, S, Wendtner C, Falk MH, Kurze V, Sauer H, Aydemir U, Hiddemann W. Neoadjuvant chemotherapy combined with regional hyperthermia (RHT) for locally advanced primary or recurrent high-risk adult soft-tissue sarcomas (STS) of adults: long-term results of a phase II study. Eur J Cancer 2001; 37(13):1599-1608.

21. Issels RD, Lindner LH, Verweij J, Wust P, Reichardt P, Schem BC, Abdel-Rahman S, Daugaard S, Salat C, Wendtner CM, Vujaskovic Z, Wessalowski R, Jauch KW, Dürr HR, Ploner F, Baur-Melnyk A, Mansmann U, Hiddemann W, Blay JY, Hohenberger P. Neo-adjuvant chemotherapy alone or with regional hyperthermia for localised high-risk soft-tissue sarcoma: a randomised phase 3 multicentrestudy. Lancet Oncol 2010;11(6):561-570.

22. Issels, RD, Lindner, LH, Verweij J, Wessalowski, R, Reichardt, P, Wust, P, Ghadjar, P, Hohenberger, P, Angele, M, Salat, C, Vujaskovic, Z, Daugaard, S, Mella, O, Mansmann, U, Dürr, HR, Knösel, T, Abdel-Rahman, S, Schmidt, M, Hiddemann, W, Jauch, KW, Belka, C, Gronchi, A. Effect of neoadjuvant chemotherapy plus regional hyperthermia on long-term outcomes among patients with localized high-risk soft tissue sarcoma: the eortc 62961-esho 95 randomized clinical trial. JAMA Oncol 2018;4(4):483-492.

23. Romanowski R, Schött C, Issels R, Klingebiel T, Treuner J, Jürgens H, Göbel U, Goldschmitt-Wuttge B, Feldmann H, Haas R. Regional hyperthermia with systemic chemotherapy in children and adolescents: feasibility and clinical follow-up of 34 intensively pretreated patients with prognostically unfavorable tumor diseases. Klin Pädiatr 1993;205(4):249-256.

24. Wessalowski R, Schneider DT, Mils O, Friemann V, Kyrillopoulou O, Schaper J, Matuschek C, Rothe K, Leuschner I, Willers R, Schönberger S, Göbel U, Calaminus G; MAKEI study group. Regional deep hyperthermia for salvage treatment of children and adolescents with refractory or recurrent non-testicular malignant germ-cell tumours: an open-label, non-randomised, single-institution, phase 2 study. Lancet Oncol 2013;14(9):843-852.

25. Van der Zee J, González González D, van Rhoon GC, van Dijk JD, van Putten WL, Hart AA. Lancet. Comparison of radiotherapy alone with radiotherapy plus hyperthermia in locally advanced pelvic tumours: a prospective, randomised, multicentre trial. Dutch Deep Hyperthermia Group 2000;355(9210):1119-1125.

26. Wust P, Hildebrandt B, Sreenivasa G, Rau B, Gellermann J, Riess H, Felix R, Schlag PM. Hyperthermia in combined treatment of cancer. Lancet Oncol 2002;3(8): 487-497.

27. Kok HP, Kotte ANTJ, Crezee J. Planning, optimisation and evaluation of hyperthermia treatments. Int J Hyperthermia 2017;33(6):593-607.

28. Paulides MM, Rodrigues DB, Bellizzi GG, Sumser K, Curto S, Neufeld E, Montanaro H, Kok HP, Dobsicek Trefna H. ESHO benchmarks for computational modeling and optimization in hyperthermia therapy. Int J Hyperthermia 2021;38(1):1425-1442.

29. Curto S, Mulder HT, Aklan B, Mils O, Schmidt M, Lamprecht U, Peller M, Wessalowski R, Lindner LH, Fietkau R, Zips D, van Holthe N, Franckena M, Paulides MM, van Rhoon GC. A multi-institution study: comparison of the heating patterns of five different MR-guided deep hyperthermia systems using an anthropomorphic phantom. Int J Hyperthermia 2020;37(1):1103-1115.

30. Stehlin JS Jr. Hyperthermic perfusion with chemotherapy for cancers of the extremities. Surg Gynecol Obstet 1969;129(2):305-8.

31. Eggermont AM, ten Hagen TL. Tumor necrosis factor-based isolated limb perfusion for soft tissue sarcoma and melanoma: ten years of successful antivascular therapy. Curr Oncol Rep 2003;5(2):79-80.

32. Sugarbaker PH, Averbach AM, Jacquet P, Stuart OA, Stephens AD: Hyperthermic intra-operative intraperitoneal chemotherapy(HIPEC) with mitomycin C. Surg Technol Int 1996;5:245–249.

33.Auer RC,Sivajohanathan D, Biagi, Conner J, Kennedy E, May T. Indications for hyperthermic intraperitoneal chemotherapy with cytoreductive surgery: A systematic review. Eur J Cancer 2020;127:76-95.

34. Deroose JP, Grünhagen DJ, de Wilt JH, Eggermont AM, Verhoef C. Treatment modifications in tumour necrosis factor-α (TNF)-based isolated limb perfusion in patients with advanced extremity soft tissue sarcomas. Eur J Cancer 2015;51(3):367-73.

35. Baas PC, Hoekstra HJ, Schraffordt Koops H, Oosterhuis JW, Oldhoff J. Isolated regional perfusion in the treatment of subungual melanoma. Arch Surg 1989; 124(3):373-376.

36. Hohenberger P, Tunn PU. Isolated limb perfusion with rhTNF-alpha and melphalan for locally recurrent childhood synovial sarcoma of the limb. J Pediatr Hematol Oncol 2003;25(11):905-990.

37. Hayes-Jordan A, Green H, Fitzgerald N, Xiao L, Anderson P. Novel treatment for desmoplastic small round cell tumor: hyperthermic intraperitoneal perfusion. J Pediatr Surg 2010;45(5):1000-1006.

38. Hayes-Jordan AA, Coakley BA., Green HL, Xiao L, Fournier KF, Herzog CE, Ludwig A, McAleer MF, Anderson PM, Huh WW. Desmoplastic small round cell

tumor treated with cytoreductive surgery and hyperthermic intraperitonealchemotherapy: results of a phase 2 trial. Ann Surg Oncol 2018;25:872-877.

39. Gesche J, Beckert S, Neunhoeffer F, Kachanov D, Konigsrainer A, Seitz G, Fuchs J. Cytoreductive surgery and hyperthermicintraperitoneal chemotherapy: A safe treatment option for intraperitoneal rhabdomyosarcoma in children below 5 years of age. Pediatr Blood Cancer 2019;66:e27517.

40. Multhoff G. Activation of natural killer cells by heat shock protein 70. 2002. Int J Hyperthermia 2009;25(3): 169-175.

41. Pandya MJ, Bendz H, Manzenrieder F, Noessner E, Kessler H, Buchner J, Issels RD. Interaction of human heat shock protein 70 with tumor-associated peptides. Biol Chem 2009;390(4):305-312.

42. Debes A, Oerding M, Willers R, Göbel U, Wessalowski R. Sensitization of human Ewing's tumor cells to chemotherapy and heat treatment by the bioflavonoid quercetin. Anticancer Res 2003;23(4):3359-66.

43. Asea A. HSP70: a chaperokine. Novartis Found Symp 2008;291:173-179.

44. Baselga J, Swain SM. Novel anticancer targets: revisiting ERBB2 and discovering ERBB3. Nat Rev Cancer 2009;9(7):463-475.

45. Wei Z, Zhan X, Fan L, Ye X, Yang X, Huang G, Li W, Wang J, Han X, Meng M, Ni Y, Li Q. Programmed death-ligand 1 expression and CD8+ tumor-infiltrating lymphocytes in advanced non-small cell lung cancer treated with microwave ablation and chemotherapy. Int J Hyperthermia 2018;35(1);591-598.

46. Issels RD, Noessner E, Lindner LH, Schmidt M, Albertsmeier M, Blay JY, Stutz E, Xu Y, Buecklein V, Altendorf-Hofmann A, Abdel-Rahman S, Mansmann U, von Bergwelt-Baildon M, Knoesel T. Immune infiltrates in patients with localised high-risk soft tissue sarcoma treated with neoadjuvant chemotherapy without or with regional hyperthermia: A translational research program of the EORTC 62961-ESHO 95 randomised clinical trial. Eur J Cancer 2021;158:123-132.

47. Rupp L Resag A, Potkrajcic V, Warm V, Wehner R, Jöhrens K, Bösmüller H, Eckert F, Schmitz M.Prognostic impact of the post-treatment T cell composition and spatial organization in soft tissue sarcoma patients treated with neoadjuvant hyperthermic radio(chemo) therapy. Front Immunol 2023;14:1185197.

5. Current and Future Clinical Trials

5.1. Chemotherapy and Hyperthermia

At present, we are witnessing the coming of age for regional "deep" hyperthermia (RHT, PBHT, HIPEC) as a treatment component for malignancies in general and, if combined with chemotherapy, for specific malignancies.

The EORTC-ESHO Intergroup trial for soft tissue sarcomas -the proof of concept

In Europe, clinical studies, primarily initiated by the European Society of Hyperthermic Oncology (ESHO) as the EORTC 62961-ESHO 95 Intergroup trial for high-risk soft tissue sarcomas (STS), can be considered as proof of concept in a time of evidence-based oncology, not only for the clinical benefit by adding hyperthermia to enhance outcome of chemotherapy, but also for adequate achievement of deep heating in locally advanced tumors. The study design allowed to define the relative contribution of regional hyperthermia and the effect of chemotherapy to the significant improvements in outcome. The positive results of the intergroup trial in high-risk STS are of great importance in several aspects. This is the first completed, large, randomized study where RHT combined with systemic chemotherapy has been applied as first-line treatment of a potentially curable disease, with significant impact on outcome [1, 2]. Secondly, the design of the phase III study was based on the results of two prior consecutive phase II studies [3, 4]. Besides safety, achievement of measured tumor temperature (T_{max} ≥42°C) and efficacy in terms of impressive progression-free survival rates were demonstrated, and the results of the phase II studies suggested that post-surgical hyperthermia were crucial for local control.

In summary, neoadjuvant chemotherapy combined with regional hyperthermia offers a standard treatment for high-risk STS where local control is difficult to achieve, and death may result from disease progression.

Immune infiltrates in patients with localized high-risk soft tissue sarcoma treated with neoadjuvant chemotherapy without or with regional hyperthermia: A translational research program of the EORTC 62961-ESHO 95 randomized clinical trial

The randomized trial showed improved long-term survival of patients with high-risk soft-tissue sarcoma by adding regional hyperthermia to neoadjuvant chemotherapy [2]. The late divergence of survival curves as observed in other immunotherapy trials suggested that immune effects induced in patients treated with neoadjuvant therapy may contribute to the clinical outcome [5]. There is strong preclinical evidence of innate and adaptive immune effects induced by heat [6-8]. The translational research program of the EORTC-ESHO trial included the objective of whether immune mechanisms in addition to the well-known drug synergy with hyperthermia might be involved in the therapy associated efficacy of the combined treatment. Therefore, we analyzed the immune infiltrate in biopsies of patients at baseline and/or after four cycles of neoadjuvant therapy to decipher the characteristics that may associate with clinical tumor response and survival.

TILs increased in paired second biopsies independent of treatment allocation (P<0.001). FOXP3 regulatory T cells decreased (P=0.002), and PD-L1 expression of tumors became undetectable. In the multi-variate analysis, post-treat-

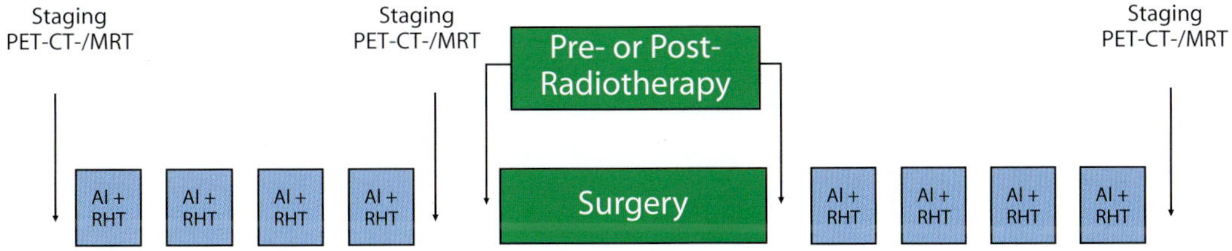

Figure 5.1: Current neoadjuvant treatment protocol at the Munich Sarcoma Center (SarKUM) for patients with high-risk soft-tissue sarcoma of adults.

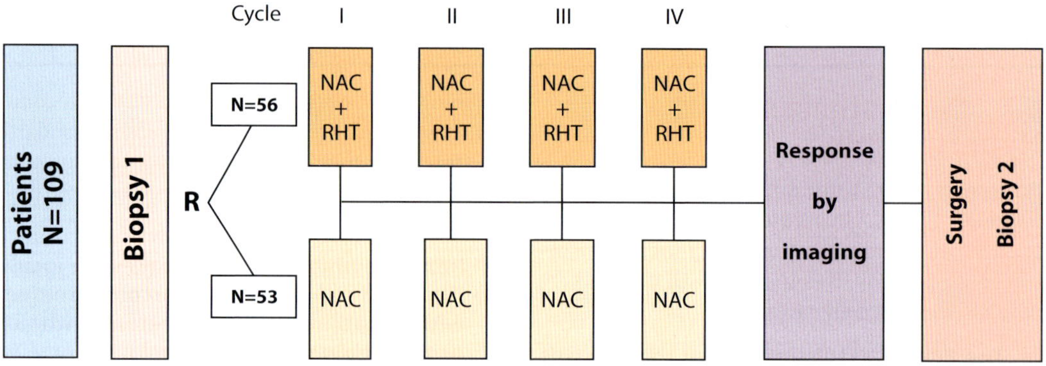

Figure 5.2A: Tumor infiltrating lymphocytes (TILs) and CD8, FOXP3, PD-1, and PD-L1 were evaluated in sequential biopsies of patients before (biopsy 1) and after four cycles of therapy (biopsy 2).

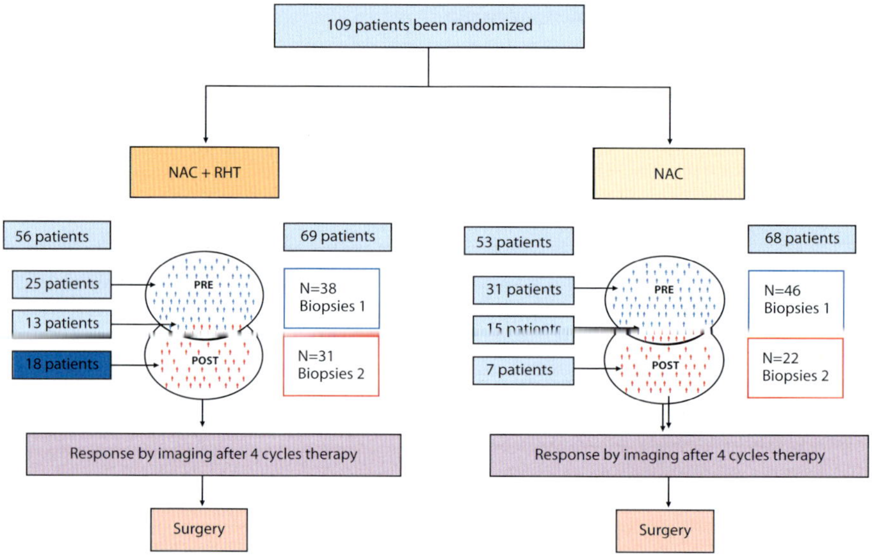

Figure 5.2B: From a subgroup of 109 patients who had been randomized between July 1997 and November 2006 to neoadjuvant chemotherapy (53 patients) or neoadjuvant chemotherapy with regional hyperthermia (56 patients), 137 biopsies were obtained.

ment high TILs correlated to LPFS (HR: 0.34; 95% CI 0.15-0.75; P=0.008) and DFS (HR: 0.38; 95% CI 0.17-0.82; P=0.015). In comparing post-treatment immune infiltrate between treatment arms with or without regional hyperthermia, tumor response was associated with neoadjuvant chemotherapy with regional hyperthermia (P=0.013) and high TILs (P=0.064). High CD8 cell infiltration was associated with improved LPFS (HR: 0.27; 95% CI 0.09-0.79; Log-rank P=0.011) and DFS (HR: 0.25; 95% CI 0.09-0.73; Log-rank P=0.006). Improved survival at 10 years was associated with immune infiltrate after neoadjuvant chemotherapy with regional hyperthermia [9].

In conclusion of the results, the preoperative therapy reprogrammed a non-inflamed tumor at baseline into an inflamed tumor. The post-treatment immune infiltrate became predictive for clinical outcomes. The combination with regional hyperthermia primes the tumor microenvironment, enabling enhanced anti-tumor immune activity in high-risk soft tissue sarcomas. The clinical results of the translational program are the basis for further immunotherapy studies in combination with regional hyperthermia. Neoadjuvant therapy induced a switch into a more inflamed tumor, which may increase the potential clinical benefit of immune checkpoint inhibitors (ICIs). Moreover, the combined treatment with regional hyperthermia led to higher tumor responses and improved survival outcomes associated with immune infiltrates of these patients. Therefore, it seems justified to consider checkpoint blockade concurrent with neo-adjuvant chemotherapy combined with regional hyperthermia as part of future trials [10]. For chemoimmunotherapy in the neo-adjuvant setting, an editorial on induction-therapy based immunological selection of patients for consecutive therapies highlighted different surrogate markers for further treatment with checkpoint inhibitors [11]. As a working hypothesis, in patients showing an objective response after four cycles of combined therapy, high CD8 infiltration in post-treatment biopsies could be used as a biomarker for continuing checkpoint blockade in these patients.

Thermosensitive Liposomes Containing Chemotherapeutic Agents – Future Clinical Aspects

Heating of tumor tissue to temperatures of up to 43°C using regional hyperthermia has been developed in the past decades as an established and efficacious treatment modality in combination with chemo- and radiotherapy. Hyperthermia can be used to further improve liposomal encapsulated chemotherapy in two ways: Hyperthermia is known to increase vascular permeability in solid tumors and may therefore increase levels of liposome accumulation, and thermosensitive liposomes have been developed that can be triggered to release their contents upon hyperthermia. By applying these two strategies, drug delivery to tumors can be strongly enhanced [12-14].

In summary, the results of phase II and phase III clinical trials, supported by a wealth of new biological data, strengthen the current evidence that hyperthermia in combination with chemotherapy is an effective and useful modality that should be integrated into the treatment of cancer (☞ Section 3.2). The conduct of randomized clinical trials is limited due to the enormous costs and regulatory hurdles to initiating and conducting RCTs without funding. There is a need for greater promotion of interest among medical oncologists and funding of RCTs by the pharmaceutical industry. Given the resources and personnel activities required for hyperthermia as a technologically safe and effective treatment modality in routine clinical practice, it is evident that reimbursement of hyperthermia by health authorities is critical. This support should be given to a qualified number of dedicated centers working in collaboration with the European Society of Hyperthermic Oncology and identified and promoted within the European community, and most importantly, their necessary support should be secured.

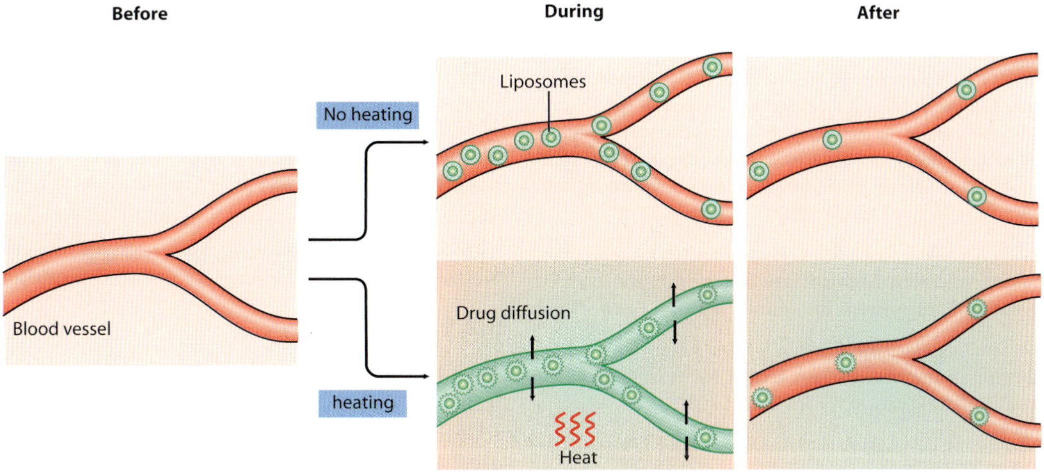

Figure 5.3: Transport of drugs encapsulated within thermosensitive liposomes from blood vessels to tumors [15].

5.1.1. References

1. Issels RD, Lindner LH, Verweij J, et al. Neo-adjuvant chemotherapy alone or with regional hyperthermia for localised high-risk soft-tissue sarcoma: a randomised phase 3 multicentre study. Lancet Oncol 2010.

2. Issels RD, Lindner LH, Verweij J, et al. Effect of neo-adjuvant chemotherapy plus regional hyperthermia on long-term outcomes among patients with localized high-risk soft tissue sarcoma: The EORTC 62961-ESHO 95 Randomized Clinical Trial. JAMA Oncol 2018.

3. Issels RD, Prenninger SW, Nagele A, et al. Ifosfamide plus etoposide combined with regional hyperthermia in patients with locally advanced sarcomas: a phase II study. J Clin Oncol 1990.

4. Issels RD, Abdel-Rahman S, Wendtner C, et al. Neo-adjuvant chemotherapy combined with regional hyperthermia (RHT) for locally advanced primary or recurrent high-risk adult soft-tissue sarcomas (STS) of adults: long-term results of a phase II study. Eur J Cancer 2001.

5. Thorén FB, Anderson H, Strannegård Ö. Late divergence of survival curves in cancer immunotherapy trials: interpretation and implications. Cancer Immunol Immunother 2013.

6. Chen T, Guo J, Han C, Yang M, Cao X. Heat shock protein 70, released from heat-stressed tumor cells, initiates antitumor immunity by inducing tumor cell chemokine production and activating dendritic cells via TLR4 pathway. J Immunol 2009.

7. Frey B, Weiss E-M, Rubner Y, et al. Old and new facts about hyperthermia-induced modulations of the immune system. Int J Hyperthermia 2012.

8. Toraya-Brown S, Fiering S. Local tumour hyperthermia as immunotherapy for metastatic cancer. Int J Hyperthermia 2014.

9. Issels RD, Noessner E, Lindner LH, et al. Immune infiltrates in patients with localised high-risk soft tissue sarcoma treated with neoadjuvant chemotherapy without or with regional hyperthermia: A translational research program of the EORTC 62961-ESHO 95 randomised clinical trial. Eur J Cancer 2021.

10. Li Z, Deng J, Sun J, Ma Y. Hyperthermia targeting the tumor microenvironment facilitates immune checkpoint inhibitors. Front Immunol 2020.

11. Shu CA, Cascone T. What Is Neo? Chemoimmunotherapy in the neoadjuvant setting for resectable non-small-cell lung cancer. J Clin Oncol 2021.

12. Koning GA, Eggermont AMM, Lindner LH, ten Hagen TLM. Hyperthermia and thermosensitive liposomes for improved delivery of chemotherapeutic drugs to solid tumors. Pharm Res 2010.

13. Zimmermann K, Hossann M, Hirschberger J, et al. A pilot trial of doxorubicin containing phosphatidyldiglycerol based thermosensitive liposomes in spontaneous feline soft tissue sarcoma. Int J Hyperthermia 2017.

14. Hossann M, Hirschberger J, Schmidt R, et al. A heat-activated drug-delivery platform based on phosphatidyl-(oligo)-glycerol nanocarrier for effective cancer treatment. Adv Nano Biomed Res 2021.

15. Dewhirst MW, Secomb TW. Transport of drugs from blood vessels to tumour tissue. Nat Rev Cancer 2017.

5.2. Radiotherapy / Chemoradiation and Hyperthermia

Most of the successful clinical hyperthermia trials of the past examined the combination of radiotherapy and hyperthermia in comparison to radiotherapy alone. Recently, the focus has been directed on the interaction of hyperthermia with chemoradiation protocols. Local and regional hyperthermia treatments are proven potent radiosensitizers in various clinical settings. However, many questions remain open. Which patients (diagnosis, tumor stage, and standard treatment) will have the biggest benefit from additional hyperthermia in combination with radiotherapy or chemoradiation? How about the combination with modern immunotherapy approaches? Although the proof of principle for the effectiveness of additional hyperthermia is no longer questionable, further studies are needed to optimize treatment schedules and patient selection criteria for the biggest clinical benefit.

Although there are numerous prospective institutional trials running in various departments all over the world, in this chapter the focus lies on running or developing studies with a multicentric design. The following studies were discussed, developed and initiated by the members of the Atzelsberg Circle (in German "Atzelberger Kreis"; web: www.atzelsbergerkreis.de), the clinical studies working group of the European Society of Hyperthermic Oncology (ESHO; web: www.esho.info).

5.2.1. Anal Cancer

The first trial addresses patients with anal cancer. Standard therapy is definitive chemoradiation with concurrent 5-FU and mitomycin C. In 2005, a small randomized Greek phase II trial showed a significant benefit for patients with anal carcinoma who received additional endoluminal hyper-

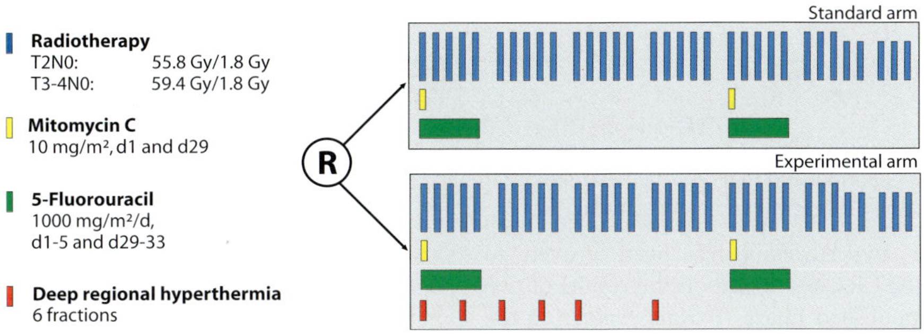

Figure 5.4: Randomized phase II trial of chemoradiation with and without deep regional hyperthermia in anal cancer.

thermia [1]. The colostomy rate at five years was 95% versus 68% in favor of the hyperthermia group. Encouraged by these results, a randomized phase II trial of chemoradiation with and without deep regional hyperthermia in anal cancer was initiated in 2014 (HyCAN trial). Eight study centers from Germany, Switzerland and Italy are participating and patient recruitment is expected to be complete in 2024. More details on this trial and the role of hyperthermia in anal cancer may be found in Chapter 3.4.4.

5.2.2. Soft Tissue Sarcoma

In perspective, another planned study will focus on soft tissue sarcoma of the extremities and trunk. In the EORTC 62961-ESHO95 trial by Issels et al., the application of 4 cycles of neoadjuvant chemotherapy in combination with hyperthermia was associated with improved survival, while only half of the patients were able to receive additional four cycles of adjuvant treatment in a randomized phase III trial [2, 3]. This highlights the need to further investigate extended neoadjuvant concepts integrating deep hyperthermia. In addition to switching from systemically effective six cycles of chemotherapy along with hyperthermia to a fully neoadjuvant approach, clinical research is focused on integrating radiation therapy into such an approach. In this context, it was shown by Semrau et al. [4] that the combination of simultaneous radiochemotherapy with hyperthermia is not only feasible with regard to subsequent surgical morbidity, but also leads to deeper pathological remissions than radiochemotherapy alone. This makes both concepts interesting for high-risk sarcomas as defined by the Sarculator (web: www.sarculator.com) with high metastatic probability but also for critically R0 resectable tumors. In this planned randomized phase II/III trial both concepts will be compared.

5.2.3. Rectal Cancer

In 2021, two randomized phase III trials have established a neoadjuvant approach called *total neoadjuvant therapy (TNT:* preoperative radiotherapy/chemoradiation and consolidation chemotherapy followed by surgery) as a new standard of care for patients with locally advanced rectal cancer UICC stage 2 and 3 [5, 6]. Besides other results, the complete remission (CR) rate increased to about 30% of the patients treated with TNT. A high CR rate is a prerequisite to introduce organ preservation strategies in patients with locally advanced rectal cancer. As already shown in Chapter 3.4.2,

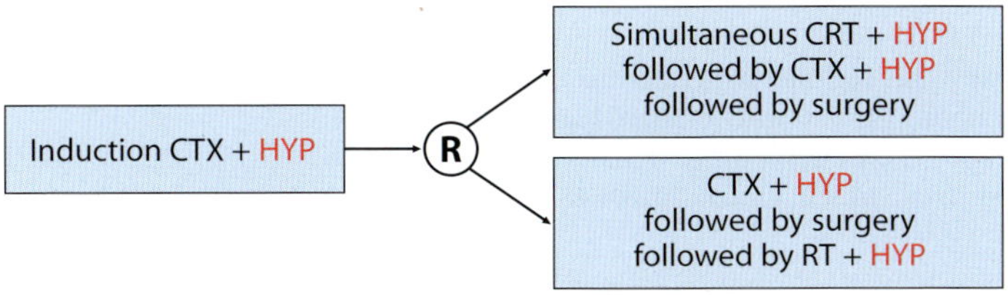

Figure 5.5: Planned randomized phase II/III trialof optimized neoadjuvant therapy concepts for high-risk soft tissue sarcomas of the extremities and trunk: Extended chemotherapy (CTX) in combination with hyperthermia (HYP) and postoperative radiation (RT) versus total neoadjuvant therapy (TNT) with concurrent chemo-radiothermotherapy (CRT+HYP followed by CTX+HYP).

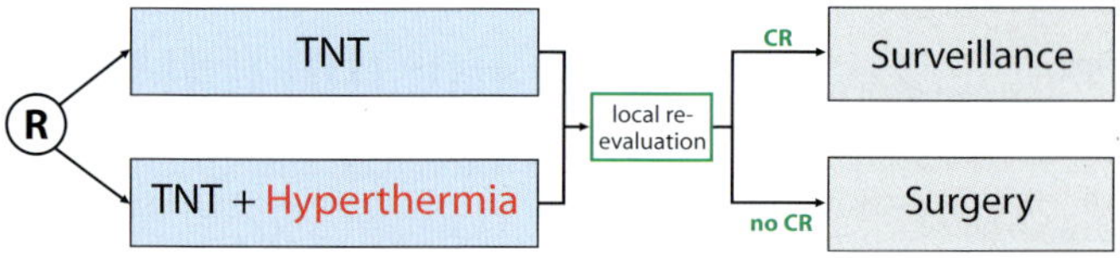

Figure 5.6: Randomized trial on total neoadjuvant therapy (TNT) with and without additional hyperthermia in patients with locally advanced rectal cancer.

additional hyperthermia has been proven to increase the CR rates. Based on the results of two recently published phase II trials evaluating the combination of chemoradiation and additional deep regional hyperthermia in locally advanced and locally recurrent rectal cancer [7, 8], efforts were made to develop a randomized phase III trial. The hypothesis of the planned trial is that additional hyperthermia may lead to higher CR rates, resulting in a higher proportion of patients who can omit mutilating surgery and enter a surveillance protocol.

Summary

The ongoing development of new clinical hyperthermia trials is essential in the context of changing standards for oncological therapies. The implementation of new clinical trials will be the only way that patients may benefit in the future from the additional radio- and chemosensitizing effects of local and regional hyperthermia treatments.

5.2.4. References

1. Kouloulias V, Plataniotis G, Kouvaris J, et al. Chemoradiotherapy combined with intracavitary hyperthermia for anal cancer: feasibility and long-term results from a phase II randomized trial. Am J Clin Oncol 2005;28:91-99.

2. Issels RD, Lindner LH, Verweij J, et al.Neo-adjuvant chemotherapy alone or with regional hyperthermia for localised high-risk soft-tissue sarcoma: a randomised phase 3 multicentre study. Lancet Oncol 2010;11(6): 561-70.

3. Issels RD, Lindner LH, Verweij J, et al. Effect of neoadjuvant chemotherapy plus regional hyperthermia on long-term outcomes among patients with localized high-risk soft tissue sarcoma: The EORTC 62961-ESHO 95 Randomized Clinical Trial. JAMA Oncol 2018;4:483-492.

4. Willner A, Agaimy A, Fechner K, et al. Chemoradiotherapy plus hyperthermia (CRTH) versus chemoradiotherapy (CRT) alone in neoadjuvant treatment of soft tissue sarcoma: tumor response, treatment toxicity and disease control. Int J Hyperthermia 2023, in press

5. Bahadoer RR, Dijkstra EA, van Etten B, et al. Short-course radiotherapy followed by chemotherapy before total mesorectal excision (TME) versus preoperative chemoradiotherapy, TME, and optional adjuvant chemotherapy in locally advanced rectal cancer (RAPIDO): a randomised, open-label, phase 3 trial. Lancet Oncol 2021;22:29-42.

6. Conroy T, Bosset J-F, Etienne P-L, et al. Neoadjuvant chemotherapy with FOLFIRINOX and preoperative chemoradiotherapy for patients with locally advanced rectal cancer (UNICANCER-PRODIGE 23): a multicentre, randomised, open-label, phase 3 trial. Lancet Oncol 2021;22:702-715.

7. Gani C, Lamprecht U, Ziegler A, et al. Deep regional hyperthermia with preoperative radiochemotherapy in locally advanced rectal cancer, a prospective phase II trial. Radiother Oncol 2021;159:155–6.

8. Ott OJ, Gani C, Lindner LH, et al. Neoadjuvant chemoradiation combined with regional hyperthermia in locally advanced or recurrent rectal cancer. Cancers (Basel) 2021;13(6):1279.

6. Summary

Quality-assured local and regional hyperthermia procedures have been proven to enhance the clinical benefits of oncological standard treatments in several clinical settings, without a significant increase in late toxicity. This makes hyperthermia an attractive sensitizer for both radiotherapy and chemotherapy. It is no longer a question whether hyperthermia is an effective oncological treatment at all. Today, the question is which patients, which tumor entity, and which clinical stage of disease will benefit the most from the addition of hyperthermia as an integral part of current multimodality oncological treatment schedules. Significant advances have been made during the past decade on the use of hyperthermia in the treatment of many cancers; e.g., cervical cancer, soft tissue sarcoma, rectal cancer, and others, but still there is a lot of work to do in the context of clinical trials in order to identify proper patient selection guidelines and to design complex multimodality treatment strategies that make the beneficial clinical effects of hyperthermia accessible for many patients.

During the past ten years technical improvements have led to better heat delivery to the tumor bearing tissue, even in deep seated malignancies in the abdomen and pelvis. Computertomography- or MRI-based individual preplanning of hyperthermia allows an optimized heat distribution with temperature maxima in the tumor and avoidance of dose limiting "hot spots" in the normal tissue, which is a prerequisite for patient compliance. With the use of non-invasive MRI-thermometry during the regional hyperthermia treatment, the pre-calculated adjustments and the consecutive heat distribution in the patient can be verified and documented.

More and more, the medical insurance companies are aware of the benefits of quality-assured local and regional hyperthermia techniques and reimburse heat applications in dedicated medical centers of excellence; e.g., in Germany, Switzerland and the Netherlands.

We hope that this booklet has opened the eyes of the interested reader to this growing field of oncology. Further information on treatment centers and clinical trials is available on the homepages of the European Society of Hyperthermic Oncology (ESHO, www.esho.info) and the Atzelsberg Circle (www.atzelsbergerkreis.de), the clinical committee of ESHO and a working group of the German Cancer Society.

Index

T

U

V